The Instructional Media Library

Volume Number 16

VIDEODISCS

Edward W. Schneider
Junius L. Bennion

with Illustrations by
Don Seegmiller

David O. McKay Institute
Brigham Young University

James E. Duane
Series Editor

Educational Technology Publications
Englewood Cliffs, New Jersey 07632

This book is a product of the Videodisc Research Project, David O. McKay Institute, Brigham Young University.

Library of Congress Cataloging in Publication Data

Schneider, Edward W
    Videodiscs.

        (The Instructional media library ; v. no. 16)
        Bibliography: p.
        1. Video discs in education. I. Bennion, Junius, L.,
joint author. II. Title. III. Series: Instructional
media library ; v. no. 16.
LB1044.7.S2785   371.3'3   80-23563
ISBN 0-87778-176-1

Copyright © 1981 Educational Technology Publications, Inc., Englewood Cliffs, New Jersey 07632.

Printed in the United States of America.

Library of Congress Catalog Card Number:
80-23563

International Standard Book Number:
0-87778-176-1

First Printing: January, 1981.

Preface

The topic of videodiscs is so multi-faceted and is changing so rapidly that additional chapters to this book could be written every three months. The chapters in your hands present the rudiments of the technology, but even some of the "basic facts" change, as new technical advances are introduced and new applications and markets are opened up. Before making any irreversible decisions, it would be wise to check on current conditions by consulting manufacturers' representatives and the latest trade journals.

The chapters in this book are as follows:

Chapter 1 describes the basic concept of the videodisc and its technology.

Chapters 2 and 3 discuss the types of educational applications that have been developed and the situational variables favoring the use of videodiscs.

Chapter 4 looks at the economics of videodiscs as compared to the economics of alternative media. The relationships that emerge illustrate the fundamental differences between videodiscs and other motion media, and justify, we believe, our optimism about the future of videodiscs.

Chapter 5 describes the processes of mastering and replicating discs.

Chapter 6 is devoted to the special features of the industrial/educational model players and the methods used to program their operation.

Chapter 7 discusses the advantages of connecting the industrial/educational players to external computer systems and the methods used to develop individualized instructional modules for these more complex systems.

Chapter 8 is our attempt to predict the direction of future developments. We don't mind prophesying, but putting such things down on paper is making us just a bit nervous! So much will happen in this area in the next ten years that this attempt to circumscribe the implications for education and training will seem very timid and narrow to future readers.

EWS
JLB
August, 1980

Acknowledgments

Many people have been part of this effort, helping us to gather together and present the facets of a new and promising technology. Without slighting the importance of their generous cooperation, we hope they will understand when we name just a few very special people who helped us to see a much larger vision than the nuts and bolts of the players and the shiny plastic of the discs:

Klaus Compaan, Philips Electro-Acoustics Division
Eddy Zwaneveld, Consolidated Film Industries
Kipp Pritzlaff, Techno-Products
Kent Broadbent, MCA DiscoVision
Georges Broussaud, Thomson-CSF
Alfred Bork, University of California, Irvine
Joseph Lipson, National Science Foundation

Table of Contents

VIDEODISCS

1.

What Is a Videodisc? How Does It Work?

A videodisc is a non-volatile storage medium for television signals, audio signals, and digital signals. It looks like a long-playing audio record that has had its grooves scraped off; the video "grooves" are so tightly packed that they are imperceptible to the naked eye.

Videodisc technology as a new communications medium was developed in the 1960s and early 1970s and was first demonstrated in the United States in 1971. It is now possible to store 60 minutes of video (or 54,000 still frames) on one side of a 12-inch videodisc.

When compared to the technology for storing audio signals, the videodisc is indeed a remarkable achievement. Of course, we have had audiodisc technology for over 75 years, and the many improvements in audio recording and playback technology, as well as in electronic circuitry, have achieved high-fidelity storage and reproduction of audio signals. The frequency range, however, of high-fidelity audio (20 to 20,000 cycles per second), as compared to the four million cycle bandwidth needed to store video signals, provides only one comparison of the differences between these two technologies. Audio records, first designed to rotate at 78 rpm, then at 45 rpm, and finally at 33 rpm, are extremely slow when compared to videodiscs, which rotate at 450 to 1,800 rpm. Because videodiscs rotate up to 55 times faster than audiodiscs, they require a much greater track density in order to store 30 minutes of program in the same area on a 12-inch disc. Videodiscs have about 18,000 tracks per radial inch, as compared to only 300 tracks per radial inch on audiodiscs; Figure 1 makes this comparison visually. Video-discs are 60 times denser in tracks per radial inch and 7.4 times denser in information per revolution.

Historically, videodisc prototypes grew out of the research efforts that led to the first commercially practical video recorders, developed in the mid-1950s. These recorders used magnetic tape, but in order to record the much higher frequencies needed to handle video signals, new techniques were developed. First was a video recorder using two-inch-wide tape with a rotating head (Snyder, 1957) that recorded video signals at right angles to the tape direction. This arrangement allowed fast head velocities but required a bulky tape drive mechanism.

A later development in recording technology used heli-cally-wrapped tape passing around a rotating recording head (see Figure 2). This arrangement also provided sufficient head velocities, utilizing a diagonal track on the tape, but still allowing the actual tape speed to be relatively slow. New materials and production techniques for both recording heads and magnetic tape, as well as more precise control circuits that minimize the effects of timebase errors and dropouts, have reduced tape speeds drastically. For non-broadcast systems using half-inch-wide videotape cassettes, recording times of eight hours have been achieved experimentally with a tape speed of only 1 7/8 ips. For many educational applications, the quality of the video from these new videocassette recorders (VHS and Beta formats) is adequate, and the cost of storage of video signals has been reduced dramatically in recent years.

Good though videocassettes may be, videodiscs have a number of advantages. For pre-recorded programs, videodiscs

Figure 1

Audiodisc vs. Videodisc

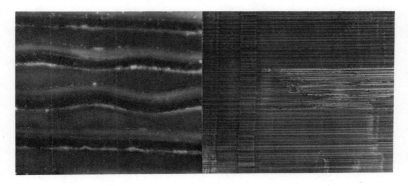

Figure 2

Closely Spaced Tracks on a Helical Videotape Recorder

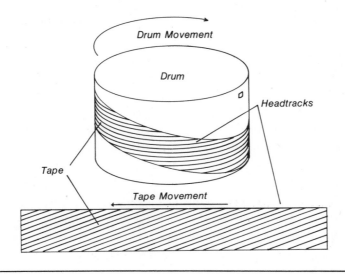

---

are cheaper and faster to replicate. Videodisc players are less expensive than all but the cheapest videotape recorders. Videodiscs are more durable than magnetic tape. They are impervious to magnetic fields and print-through. They are light-weight and easy to store or ship. Generally, the quality of videodisc images exceeds taped images in resolution, image stability, and freedom from noise. As a bonus, some videodiscs can provide random access, stop action, and slow motion under very precise computer control. Of course, not all videodisc systems are alike, as we shall soon see.

Mechanical Videodisc Systems

Videodisc systems that have a stylus or probe touching the surface of the videodisc in order to retrieve the recorded signal are termed *mechanical videodisc systems*. There are two of these types that we shall discuss. First, there is the needle-in-the-groove type, which is exemplified by the TED (*Te*lefunken/*De*cca) system (see Figure 3). The TED videodisc technology is more closely related to the audio record technology than are the other types of videodiscs. The TED videodisc, first marketed in Europe in 1974, contains ten minutes of video programming on one side of a thin, flexible, plastic disc. It was first available in the PAL (625 lines-50 cycle) television format, but later versions, produced in Japan, have used the American NTSC (525 lines-60 cycle) format. In the TED system, a sled-shaped sapphire stylus (see Figure 4) reads the grooves in the disc in a manner similar to audio record techniques, except that the grooves are much denser, and the information is recorded in the bottom of the groove, instead of in the side walls. The stylus is mounted on a relatively long pivot arm, and will continue to track for several rotations of the disc after the carriage has been stopped. The stylus will flip back and repeat short sections over and over when the carriage is stationary. As the disc wears out, the ability of the stylus to remain in the groove

Figure 3

TED Videodisc Player

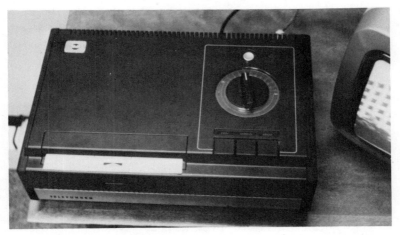

Figure 4

TED Stylus in Groove

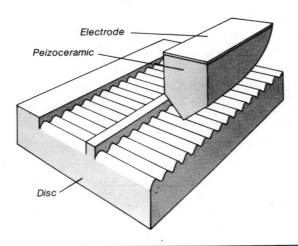

decreases, and the segment that is repeated becomes short-ened from two to three seconds to less than 1/2 second.

The second type of mechanical videodisc uses a *capacitance probe*. This is exemplified by two manufacturers: RCA and JVC (see Figures 5 and 6). The RCA system uses a diamond or a sapphire dielectric sled with a metal probe on the rear of the sled that rides in shallow U-shaped grooves on the videodisc. Changes in capacitance occur as the distance between the metal probe and the metallic layer of the disc changes (see Figure 7). The disc rotates at 450 revolutions per minute, and can hold up to one full hour of programming per side. It should last for 500 plays, and a stylus life of 1,000 hours is expected. The RCA system carries four television frames per revolution, and therefore it cannot freeze a frame or play in slow motion.

The JVC-VHD (video high density) system also uses a capacitance probe to read the videodisc, but JVC uses electronic tracking signals to maintain the position of the probe on the track (see Figure 8). This permits the disc surface to be flat and also permits the sled to be larger, thus reducing the pressure and wear to the disc and to the capacitance probe. It also allows the disc to rotate at 900 rpm, twice the speed of the RCA system.

In effect, the JVC system combines some of the features of both competing technologies (RCA and MCA/Philips-Magnavox). The electronic stylus can reread the same track to produce a still frame. However, since the disc contains two frames per revolution, a severe "jittering" of parts of the image will result during the motion scenes. Two solutions to this problem are offered by JVC. First, for purposefully designed freeze frames, they will record two identical frames on one revolution of the videodisc so that no jitter will occur on playback. Second, an auxiliary electronic "field storage" device will be available for about $150 that will digitize the video signal for one field and then provide freeze frame

Figure 5

RCA SFT 100 Videodisc Player

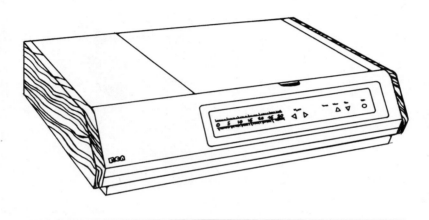

Figure 6

JVC-VHD Videodisc Player

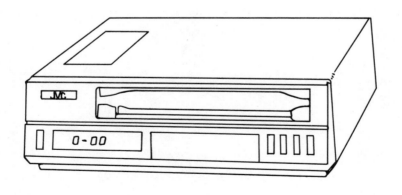

Figure 7

RCA Disc and Stylus

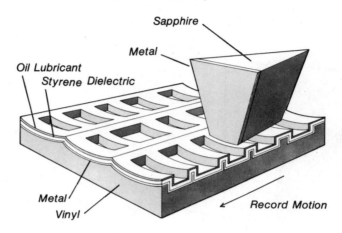

Figure 8

JVC Disc and Stylus

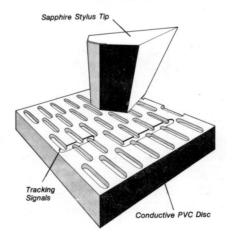

capabilities by refreshing the video signal from the storage device. In either case, the stylus continues to touch the surface of the disc when the freeze frame mode is used. Consequently, this videodisc system may not be too useful for interactive instruction, due to the wear factor on freeze frames needed for instructional components such as questions, feedback messages, segment maps, etc. For example, early reports (Roberts, 1979) indicated that the JVC system would play a videodisc 10,000 times. Although this is a significant improvement over the 50-60 plays for film or the 250+ plays for videocassettes, it is still a problem for still frames. Any still frame will receive 10,000 plays in only 11 minutes! Videodiscs designed for instructional use that are used repeatedly by many students in a learning resource center would rapidly wear out those freeze frames needed for interactive instruction. Such rapid wear-out of frames specifically designed to be viewed as still frames severely limits the use of physical-contact videodisc for interactive instruction. As a result of this limitation, we believe that both the RCA and JVC videodisc systems will be used mainly for the home entertainment market rather than for educational purposes.

Optical Videodisc Systems

Videodisc systems that use a light beam to read video, audio, and digital signals are termed *optical videodisc systems*. There are two types of optical videodisc systems: transmissive and reflective. The transmissive system (see Figure 9a) uses a clear plastic disc with a light source on one side and a light detector on the opposite side. A constant level of light from the source (usually, but not necessarily, a laser) is focused onto the videodisc through a series of mirrors and lenses so that a very small spot of light (about one micron in diameter) is formed at the surface of the videodisc. As the videodisc rotates, the intensity of the laser light is modulated by microscopic pits that have been pressed

Figure 9a

Reading a Transmissive Disc

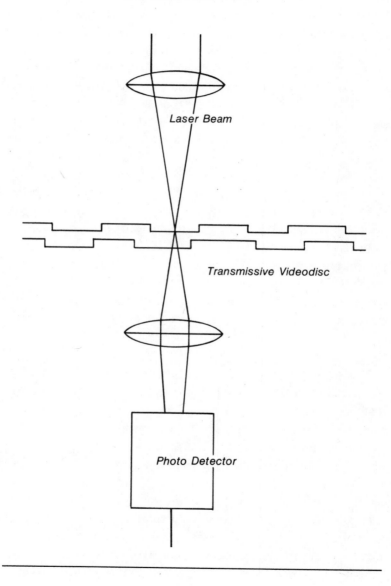

Laser Beam

Transmissive Videodisc

Photo Detector

into the plastic. The modulated light beam is then detected by a photodiode that transforms the light into an electrical signal.

The reflective videodisc system (see Figure 9b) is similar to the transmissive system, except that the light beam reflects off a shiny surface and then passes back through the same optics used to focus the laser beam onto the disc. As the disc rotates, the reflected beam is modulated by the change in distance and surface roughness between the pits and the smooth areas (the lands) between the pits. Less light is returned when the spot of light traverses a pit than when reflecting back from a land. The reflected light beam is separated from the incident beam when it passes through a beam splitter (see Figure 9c). The modulated beam is focused on a photodiode and is transformed into an electrical signal.

Figure 9b

Reading a Reflective Disc

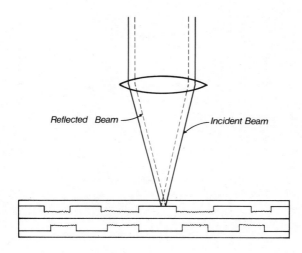

Reflected Beam —   — Incident Beam

Figure 9c

Separating Incident and Reflected Light

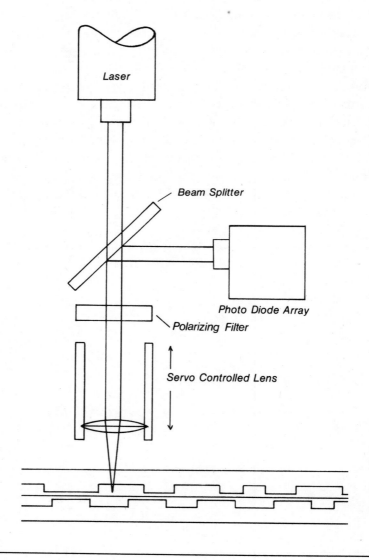

There are several differences between the transmissive and reflective optical videodisc systems. The transmissive videodisc player can read both sides of its disc by merely refocusing the optical beam of light so that it converges on the opposite surface of the disc. Thus, it is possible to retrieve twice the amount of material without having to turn the disc over in the machine. In contrast to the reflective videodisc, the transmissive disc does not have a protective plastic coat over the pits and, consequently, it must be protected from dust and fingerprints. This is done by housing the transmissive videodisc in a rigid sleeve that must be inserted into the player. When the sleeve is withdrawn, the player retains the disc and a supporting drawer. A spindle lock then lifts the disc away from the drawer and attaches it to the drive spindle. The disc itself is made of flexible plastic, but the rigid sleeve protects the disc, which is one of the advantages of this feature for storage and shipping.

Examples of both types of optical videodiscs are now available in the United States. The Thomson-CSF videodisc system (see Figure 10), produced in France, is the only transmissive type currently available. It sells for $3,500. The Magnavox 8000 ($775) (see Figure 11), the Pioneer VP-1000 ($749) (see Figure 12), and the DVA DiscoVision PR7820 ($3,000) (see Figure 13) videodisc systems use reflective videodiscs produced by MCA DiscoVision. In 1979, MCA sold half of its interest in videodiscs to IBM, and the partnership started a new company—DiscoVision Associates (DVA). Backing from the computer giant virtually guarantees that the technology will be made to succeed.

The optical videodisc never wears out because it is "read" with a light beam. For the same reason, the light beam can be moved across the spinning disc at various speeds and directions without damaging the disc. If the movement of the beam is properly synchronized with the rotation of the disc, a stable television image is produced. If the NTSC television

Figure 10

Thomson-CSF TTV3620 Videodisc Player

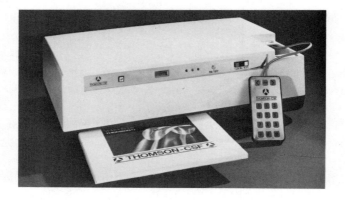

Photo: Thomson-CSF

Figure 11

Magnavox 8000 Videodisc Player

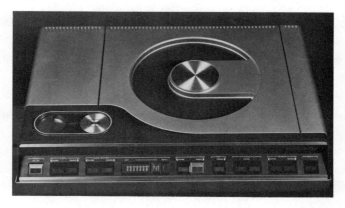

Photo: North American Philips Corp.

Figure 12

Pioneer VP-1000 "LaserDisc"

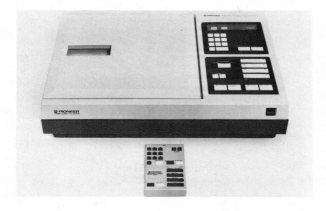

Photo: U.S. Pioneer Electronics Corp.

Figure 13

DiscoVision Associates PR7820 Videodisc Player

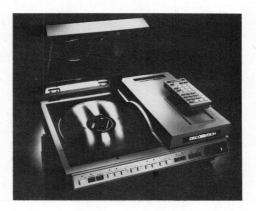

Photo: DiscoVision Associates

---

format is used, the beam must read 30 frames per second. If the beam reads consecutive frames at this rate, a normal motion sequence results. If the beam reads the same frame 30 times per second, a freeze frame results. Slow motion can be produced by reading each frame several times before moving on to the next one. To be able to switch back and forth between frames without losing synchronization, the frames must be formatted on the disc so that, as the track of pits spirals out from the center of the disc, the start of each frame is located on a common radius. This format is called Constant Angular Velocity (CAV), because the disc rotates through a constant angular displacement per unit of time: 30 revolutions per second (see Figures 14a and 14b).

Figure 14a illustrates the CAV format, and contrasts it with the Constant Linear Velocity (CLV) format (see Figure 14b). With CLV, a constant length of the spiral track passes the light beam each second, roughly 31.4 feet per second. As the circumference of the track increases, the spindle motor slows down to maintain the same linear velocity. At the outside diameter of the disc, the spindle is turning at ten revolutions per second. By reducing the average rotational speed, the CLV format can pack up to twice as much program on a disc, but it does so at the expense of freeze-frame and slow-motion capabilities. These motion-control features, along with the digital frame addresses, are important for instructional developers because they permit new instructional strategies. For example:

> It is critically important to recognize that videodisc systems can easily allow for a "mixed access" combination of single-frame and normal-time playback. The player can move easily from freeze to motion and back, either manually or automatically, and the sequence may be either programmed into the disc or controlled externally.
>
> If you are a program designer who plans to use the videodisc as an instruction and training medium, you start with a "budget" of 54,000 frames, and you can employ

Figure 14a

Format of Constant Angular Velocity (CAV) Disc

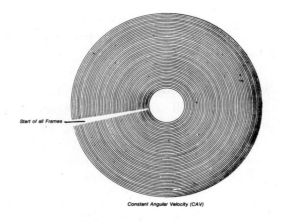

Constant Angular Velocity (CAV)

Figure 14b

Format of Constant Linear Velocity (CLV) Disc

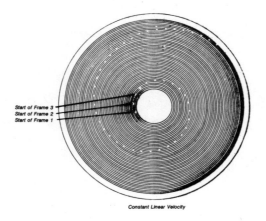

Constant Linear Velocity

them in whatever mix of still and motion sequences you
think will get the job done effectively. No more fooling
around with a closet-full of unrelated and uncoordinated
slide, film, and tape hardware. You will be able to do it all
on one medium (Winslow, 1977).

A comparison of the videodisc systems that have been
announced as of June 1, 1980 is presented in Table 1. This
Table lists seven videodisc systems and provides comparisons
for several items of interest. Although the TED system is not
being marketed in the United States, it is listed because of its
historical significance. Of the videodisc players designed for
the consumer market, the JVC-VHD, the Magnavox Model
8000, and the Pioneer VP-1000 are capable of almost the
same type of special effects. The Thomson-CSF TTV3620
player, designed and marketed for institutional use, has a
two-times feature (2X) that doubles the normal motion rate.

Note that the reflective optical players will all play the
same disc, while the other players are mutually incompatible.

Table 1

Videodisc Systems—Mid-1980 Status

MANUFACTURER	TELEFUNKEN/ DECCA	RCA
Model Name/#	TED	SelectaVision SFT 100
Market	Consumer	Consumer
Market Date	1974 (PAL)	1981
Cost of Player	$400	$500 (?)
Playback Type	Mechanical	Mechanical
Playback System	Peizo electric stylus	Capacitance probe
Tracking Method	Stylus in groove	Stylus in groove
Special Effects Controls	Repeat short segments	(None)
Remote Controller	(None)	(None)
Disc Rotation Rate (rpm)	1,500 (PAL) 1,800 (NTSC)	450
Playing Time/Side	10 min.	60 min.
Media Packaging	Protective sleeve	Protective caddy
Number of Audio Tracks	1	1
Compatibility Code	A	B
Cost—per Disc —per 2hr. Pgm.*	No U.S. Market	$5 $20

*Based on commercially available programming.

Table 1 (Continued)

JAPAN VICTOR CO. (JVC)	MAGNAVOX (PHILIPS)	PIONEER
JVC-VHD	Magnavision Model 8000	Laserdisc VP-1000
Consumer	Consumer	Consumer
1981	1978	1981
$500 (?)	$775	$750
Mechanical	Optical	Optical
Capacitance probe	Laser	Laser
Electronic servo with accessory ($150)	Electro-optical servo	Electro-optical servo
Still, slow motion Visual scan	Still, slow motion 3X*, visual scan	Still, slow motion 3X*, visual scan
(None)	(None)	Optional ($50)
900	1,800	1,800
60 min.	30 min. (CAV) 60 min. (CLV)	30 min. (CAV) 60 min. (CLV)
Protective caddy	Can be handled	Can be handled
2	2	2
C	D	D
$5 $20	$6 $25	$6 $25

*3X = Plays 3 times normal playing speed.
CAV = Constant Angular Velocity
CLV = Constant Linear Velocity

Table 1 (Continued)

DISCOVISION ASSOCIATES	THOMSON-CSF
PR7820	TTV3620
Industrial; Educational	Institutional
1979	1978
$3,000	$3,000
Optical	Optical
Laser	Laser
Electro-optical servo	Electro-optical servo
Still, slow motion programmable frame search, computer	Still, slow motion frame search, computer 2X*
Programmable (see Figure 24)	Not programmable (see Figure 25)
1,800	1,500 (PAL) 1,800 (NTSC)
30 min. (CAV) 60 min. (CLV)	30 min.**
Can be handled	Protective caddy
2	2
D	E
$6 $25	No catalog Industrial use only

*2X = Plays 2 times normal playing speed.
**Can play both 30 min. sides without manual intervention.

2.

Some Considerations in the Design of Videodisc Applications

Whether or not to use videodiscs for a particular application is a relative question—it is relative to the other available media that might be used to do the same job. Comparisons between alternative media must include the costs, capabilities, capacities, etc., of each system, properly weighted for the needs of the particular instructional situation. Next, the advantages and disadvantages must be "traded-off" to select the best alternative. This is not a matter of simply lining up specification sheets and scoring the devices feature by feature. Other factors must also be considered: historical usage patterns, availability, maintainability, durability of the program materials, compatibility with the physical and operational characteristics of the instructional environment, etc.

In his excellent book titled *How to Read a Film*, James Monaco prepared a table which compares a wide variety of media in terms of their use as channels of communication between a producer and the public. That table is reproduced as Table 2. The "Media Economics" columns answer the question, "What motivates the development of this medium?" The "Media Politics" columns describe the type of communication system that each medium represents. In his discussion of the table, Monaco comments:

Table 2

General Characteristics of Various Media
(from *How to Read a Film*, with permission)

| MEDIUM | MEDIA ECONOMICS | | MEDIA POLITICS | | | | |
	NEXUS	SALES ORIENTATION	CHANNELS	ACCESS	INTERACTION	DISTRIBUTION FLOW	CONSUMER CONTROL
books	distribution	object	open	good	unidirectional	discrete	yes
newspapers & magazines	prod./dist.	object, ad space, audience	open	good	unidirectional	semidiscrete mosaic	yes
film	distribution	entertainment	open	limited	unidirectional	discrete	some
radio	prod./dist.	ad time, audience	limited	limited	mainly unidir.	continuous	no
CB	manufacture	equipment	limited	excellent	interactive	continuous	no
audiodiscs	prod./dist.	object	open	fair	unidirectional	discrete	yes
audiotapes	production	object	open	good	unidirectional	discrete	yes
television	dist. (prod.)	ad time, audience	closed	none	unidirectional	continuous	no
cable	distribution	entertainment	limited	some	mainly unidir.	continuous	no
videodisc	manufacture	equipment	open	limited	unidirectional	discrete	yes
videotape	manufacture	equipment	open	good	unidirectional	discrete	yes

NEXUS: Where does the concentration of economic power lie? SALES ORIENTATION: What is the primary product being sold? CHANNELS: Are there a limited number of distribution channels? ACCESS: How easy is it for someone to gain access to the medium? INTERACTION: Is the medium unidirectional or interactive? DISTRIBUTION FLOW: Are the items distributed singly or continuously? CONSUMER CONTROL: Must the consumer/spectator/reader/listener adjust his or her schedule to that of the medium, or can he or she control the time and location of the experience? (from Monaco, 1977)

A close examination of the chart reveals some interesting facts. Physical items such as books, newspapers, magazines, records, and tapes have considerable advantage over the broadcast media. They are produced and distributed discretely, so the consumer can exercise choice more easily. The consumer also controls the experience; one can listen to a record, read a book, or watch a videodisc as frequently as one likes at whatever speed one prefers.

On the economic side, the characterization of the media seems to be highly correlated with the medium's maturity, i.e., its relative novelty and the size of its installed base of equipment. The newer media must initially concentrate on building up a large installed base. Once everyone has a television set or tape recorder, the sales volume necessarily shifts toward the distribution of materials to be used with the equipment. This was true of television and radio in their infancies, and it may well have been true of film, back in the days when the first projectors were being marketed. The MCA/Philips marketing arrangements for the home videodisc player may well be unique; one company is concerned with the manufacturing of equipment (Philips-Magnavox), while the other company is concerned primarily with the distribution of entertainment materials (MCA). If both marketing directions are pursued simultaneously, videodisc might see a much more rapid development than its predecessor media.

While Table 2 gives some general comparisons between videodisc and other media, we need to examine certain situational factors before we can decide on the appropriateness of the application. Some of these situational factors are listed in Table 3. A few comments on these factors may be helpful. One of the most obvious pluses for a videodisc application would be the availability of suitable instructional material from the commercial catalogs of the videodisc distributors. We have encountered several cases where the differential between purchasing the content in 16mm format versus purchasing it as a videodisc would just about pay for

Table 3

Situational Factors to Be Examined for
Instructional Applications of Optical Videodiscs

Favorable Factors	Unfavorable Factors
Suitable content is already available on discs.	Content (images and sound) will have to be revised frequently.
Many copies (140 or more) are needed.	Content consists of large blocks of text.
Copies will have to be shipped to widely dispersed sites.	Images require higher resolution than television screen can provide.
Content will be used repeatedly (thousands of plays per copy).	Suitable viewing facilities are not available (esp. for large groups).
Content requires thousands of still frames.	
Content requires rapid random access.	Content must be available for distribution in less than eight weeks.
Content requires slow motion and/or freeze frame for analysis of motion sequences.	Content cannot be divided into blocks of 27 minutes/48,600 video frames (reflective disc) or 55 minutes/100,000 video frames (transmissive disc).
Content requires "instant replay."	
Content is part of a larger instructional system and could benefit from integrated control via computers.	
A large amount of content must be stored in a small physical space (on board a submarine, for example).	

the videodisc player itself! We have yet to learn how many discs the RCA catalog will offer, but the initial MCA offering is about 160 discs, not all of which have been made available as of the date of this writing.

Shipping copies is a positive factor for videodisc. This has to do with the difference in weight among heavy film cans, moderately heavy videocassettes, and very light videodiscs. If the content is used in an individualized instructional situation, and will be played over and over again, there may be some advantages to transferring the content to videodisc, even though the number of copies required is less than the normal break-even point between disc and videotape. The reason for this is that videotape is good for only 250 to 300 plays, while the optical disc is insensitive to the number of times it has been played. If the content contains thousands of still frames, and cannot be shown in an entirely linear and mechanical fashion, videodisc may be justified even if only a single copy is required. A single videodisc with more than 5,477 still frames may be cheaper than duplicating the same number of 35mm mounted slides.

Among the unfavorable factors, it should be clear that if the content has to be revised frequently, each revision implies a new pressing of the videodisc. The fewer times the costly transfer process has to be invoked, the better. Similarly, if the content consists of large blocks of printed text, the resolution of the 525-line television system will preclude the display of more than approximately 700 characters at any one time. This means that a typical typewritten page would require three video frames to display the information in a readable form. A certain amount of overlap and, therefore, inefficiency will be inevitable, especially if the aspect ratio (the ratio of height to width) of the source material does not match the 1:1.33 ratio of the television image. The viewing facilities that will be available to the end-user should also influence the use of videodisc. For individual viewing, a small direct-view television set is universally acceptable, but for large groups, a room specially equipped with a number of large-screen monitors or a large-screen projection television system is required. Even then, certain presentations may lose much of their appeal when seen by a large group in a big room on many little screens.

At the present time (June, 1980), DiscoVision Associates is quoting a delivery time of 45 working days after the receipt of the materials to be transferred. For some applications, this lag between production of content and its availability for distribution may be unacceptable. Lastly, the capacity of the discs must be considered. At the present time, problems with the replication of the outside portion of reflective discs limit their capacity to 27 minutes; the content has to be gracefully divisible by some number close to 27 minutes so that it can be distributed onto the necessary number of sides. If on-line capacity is a problem, the transmissive disc may offer a solution because it can switch sides without requiring that the disc be turned over. This means having 100,000 video frames available without having to change discs.

If applications for the mechanical videodiscs are being contemplated, the easiest generalization is to think of them as audiodiscs that play video. Unless suitable content is already commercially available, we would not recommend them for educational applications, because we feel strongly that most educational applications can benefit from the durability and media manipulation that are only possible with the optical videodisc.

3.

Applications for Instruction

In the few months since videodiscs have become available for educational applications, a number of research groups have been developing discs to demonstrate videodisc capabilities in a wide variety of instructional situations. The most aggressive groups have been the University of Nebraska Videodisc Design/Production group (sponsored by the Corporation for Public Broadcasting), the Massachusetts Institute of Technology Architecture Machine group (sponsored by the Cybernetics Technology Office of the Defense Advanced Research Projects Agency), the University of Utah/WICAT, Inc. group (sponsored by the National Science Foundation), and the Utah State University group (sponsored by the U.S. Army and Control Data Corporation).

While research projects have been getting underway, videodisc technology has not been confined to the laboratory; General Motors Corporation has already installed players and television sets in over 11,000 dealerships across the country. Such rapid installation of such a large network clearly shows that the videodisc's future is no longer hypothetical.

This chapter describes only the most important applications; the ones that we feel will have the greatest impact on future instructional systems. We have no doubt slighted many first-rate productions and thriving production groups as a result of our ignorance and prejudices, so this chapter should be read as neither an exhaustive list nor an honor roll.

Group Instruction

By group instruction, we mean classroom instruction or lecture instruction. These environments are quite distinct from the large group which broadcast television reaches, which is really composed of many very small groups. In these classroom situations, television, in the form of closed-circuit television, has been used in schools for a number of years. A serious drawback to closed-circuit television is the rigidity of scheduling that it requires. Programs must start at fixed times, and classes must be ready to see them. Videodisc shares with videotape the ability for local control and scheduling; the teacher can start or stop the show any time he or she chooses. In addition, videodisc players are exceptionally quiet in operation and can be started and stopped instantly.

The videodisc branching capability can be used to some extent by employing a branching movie technique. Suppose, for example, that we wish to have a discussion on child-parent relationships. The situation could be presented and developed on the first half of the videodisc, illustrating the problem, and then the disc could be stopped while the class discusses what "ought" to happen or what will probably happen. The class could vote to express their preference or consensus on the most likely outcome. The second half of the disc would contain a series of endings, and the one selected could be viewed by moving the disc to the appropriate starting frame number.

In the final analysis, the extent to which videodisc will directly replace videotape and closed-circuit television will be determined primarily by economic factors (see Chapter 4: Videodisc Economics). The most likely exception to this conclusion is the teaching of skilled motor performances, where slow motion and stop action will greatly enhance the instructional value of conventional motion footage. For example, the Nebraska group has made a disc to teach basic tumbling skills to young gymnasts, and there is a sequence on the first Utah State disc that demonstrates the proper technique for the Leroy lettering device.

More radical applications take advantage of the videodisc's ability to search and its ability to store still frames as well as motion and sound. One of our colleagues, a professor of biology, has suggested that a series of discs be prepared to serve as "mediabases" for basic lectures in biology (or any other highly visual subject). Each disc in the series would contain a wide variety of illustrations of a particular set of concepts, such as cell differentiation or the taxonomy of the animal kingdom. Using an industrial/educational model player (see Chapter 6), the lecturer could select in advance the sequences which he or she wished to use, and pre-program the player to retrieve those sequences on demand. During the lecture, the lecturer would have complete control over a single comprehensive medium, starting and stopping it at will to add comments or to repeat a sequence in answer to student questions. The one system would replace overhead projectors, slide projectors, and film projectors. The resulting images could be viewed without turning off room lights, and transitions between live lecture and canned presentation would be much less noticeable. This is a distinct advantage over film projectors, where teachers must turn over control to the projection system, wait for the film to unwind, and then temporize while students blink and squint, as they readapt to bright room lights.

The same basic rules for using television in the classroom also apply to videodiscs, because the videodisc player is electrically equivalent to any other source of television signals, with the important difference that the viewer runs his or her own "station." For best classroom viewing, the room lights should be left on, but the television screens should be shielded from glare. The best viewing distance is between three and five times the diagonal measure of the screen, so one 21" receiver will serve a maximum of 15 to 20 students. The loudspeakers used in "portable" model receivers are too small for classroom use; an additional sound system will make the soundtrack much more realistic. If possible, the screens and seating should be arranged so that every viewer sees just one screen (Chapman, 1960; Lewis, 1961).

Some of the videodisc players have wireless remote control keyboards that transmit infra-red signals. When they are pointed directly at the player, their maximum range is approximately 7.5 meters. Over shorter distances, the signal can be bounced off light-colored walls and ceilings. If the player cannot be positioned to "see" the remote unit's signal, a miniature shielded cable can be used to connect them.

Individualized Instruction

Videodiscs really come into their own as individualized viewing devices. The ability to manipulate and control the medium implies control by one individual; why not let it be the student? Movies and filmstrips and other television materials have always been group-viewing experiences because of the costs of the materials and the complexities of equipment, set-up, and operation. If we imagine a continuum of applications between the group mode and a maximally interactive individualized mode, the first step away from the group mode would be to place a player, a TV monitor, and earphones at the back of the classroom. The quiet, simple-to-operate player and the durable discs would allow students to view discs on their own, without disturbing the rest of the class. The next step would be to use a few auto-stop codes at specially-prepared still frames. This would be done when the disc is mastered. When it is played back, the program would stop when the codes are encountered. In this way, the student can be asked questions, be shown written summaries, or be given study options. The first educational disc made by WICAT was an adaptation of two McGraw-Hill biology films that used this technique. It was designed to be played on the Magnavox home player. At any branch point, the student may also press the INDEX key twice to get chapter numbers, then press the SEARCH key to move to the start of the designated chapter. The Pioneer home player is more convenient for this sort of logic because it will search for a chapter by number, which makes it much easier to go back and repeat.

The next step on our continuum uses the programmable features of the DVA PR7820. These features are described in Chapter 6. For this discussion, it is enough to know that a program can be written to control the player, that the program can be transferred to a disc as a step in the disc mastering process, and that it can be read off the disc and stored in the player's memory whenever the disc is played. When the program is executed, the player appears to "know" how the disc is organized, and can branch to different parts of the content in response to the viewer's choice of pushbuttons.

The largest application of this technique was implemented in 1979, when General Motors Corporation ordered 11,500 industrial-model players for installation in all of its dealerships. The players are mounted on roll-around carts, with 19-inch color receivers mounted above them, and shelves for disc storage below (see Figure 15). More than 20 discs have already been released to dealers, with more on the way. The discs cover three distinct applications: (1) Training salespeople in basic selling skills such as finding prospects, listening to the customer, demonstrating the product, overcoming objections, and closing the sale. Other discs provide motivational pep talks or the technical skills needed to sell trucks. (2) Training mechanics to service new products, such as the 1980 Chevrolet Citation, or teaching them how to fix

Figure 15

General Motors Video Center

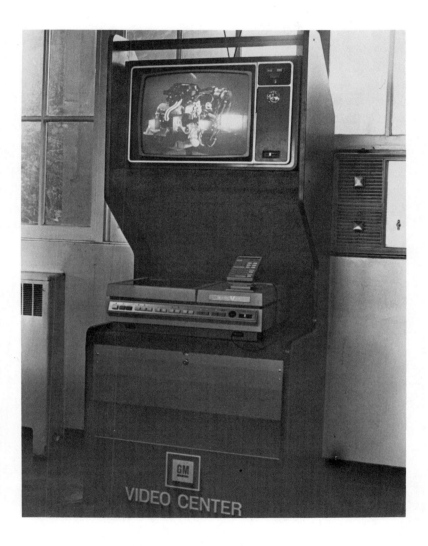

water leaks, power brakes, and four-wheel drive vehicles. (3) Making sales presentations to customers. Discs for the 1980 Buicks and for all of the Chevrolet passenger cars have been produced. Some discs in the "New Product Training Series" have three sections, one for each of these applications, to introduce a new product to the customer, salesperson, and mechanic on a single disc. On the disc covering light-duty trucks, there is a sales quiz. A still frame with a true-false or multiple-choice question is presented, the salesperson responds by pressing one of the buttons on the remote-control unit, and the player branches to the appropriate "RIGHT" or "WRONG" frame. If the answer was correct, the next question is presented. If it was incorrect, the player replays the portion of the sales presentation that answers the question, and then goes on to the next question. The dealers that we have visited have been impressed with the videodisc system, but they admit that their employees are not yet taking full advantage of it.

Further along the continuum, we see videodiscs attached to computers as part of computer-assisted instruction (CAI) systems. With videodiscs, the CAI system would not be limited to writing out messages for the student but could actually show real-world objects and happenings.

The excitement generated by the combination of the optical videodisc and microcomputers for individualized instruction is evident in the following description of these systems by Leveridge (1979):

> We know the power of audiovisual education to show what can best be learned by seeing and hearing. We know the value of interactive programs—thanks to automation by computer. But it is only through actual participation that one can fully appreciate the impact when both media are combined to deliver computer-assisted audiovisual education. It does not seem possible for words or pictures to communicate the excitement that this process generates. Even bystanders, though impressed, fail to appreciate the full flavor of the experience the participant enjoys. And, it

> is the videodisc that makes integration of the two media
> practical. By making audiovisual communication inter-
> active, the videodisc has created a new dimension in
> teaching and testing.

Still further along the continuum is a simulated world with which the student can interact.

As an example, we have proposed a method for teaching optimal control settings for metal-cutting operations. A disc could explain the nature of each of the settings (e.g., workpiece speed, feed speed, cutting angle, cutting depth, cutting tool geometry, etc.). The remainder of the disc could be devoted to a series of short clips of motion sequences, showing the cutting machine working under various combinations of settings. Any one of these clips could be viewed repeatedly, because the videodisc player would be programmed to repeat it over and over again. To give the student some practice, the videodisc player could be attached to a CAI system, and the system could select one of the motion clips at random. After viewing the clip and listening to the sound of the cutting tool, the student would indicate whether any adjustments were necessary, and if so, which ones, and in which direction the adjustment should be made. The system would find and display the clip most closely resembling the new settings, and then ask again if adjustments were needed. When the correct settings are finally obtained, the system could show the student the path that had been taken from the initial clip to the final one. The straighter the path, the better the performance.

If each student were required to make all of the set-ups that could be shown on the disc, weeks would be spent in the shop, and a lot of metal shavings would cover the floor, to say nothing of the risk of creating dangerous combinations which could fracture the cutting tools or break the machine.

In another application, videodiscs would be excellent for true-to-life automobile driving simulators. MIT has been developing a method for creating the visual database for such a system. To prepare the videodisc, cameras are mounted on a moving vehicle, and the scenes shot, one frame for every ten feet of travel, on motion picture film. One of their cameras is equipped with a very wide-angle anamorphic lens. The lens introduces distortion, but it packs a wide-angle view into the conventionally-sized frame. The resulting footage is edited onto two videodiscs in such a way that scenes can be alternated from one disc to the next. After the footage is transferred to videodisc, the simulation can begin. Pressing on a pedal varies the rate of videodisc playback; minor variations in steering correction are accomplished by shifting the image optically. This is done by laterally rotating the lens, which rectifies (i.e., optically corrects) the portion of the ana-morphic image that the student driver can see. Major changes in direction are handled by changing from one disc player to the other. For example, the voice of the driving instructor might say, "Turn right at the next intersection." If the student started to turn right, the simulator would switch from the straight-ahead scene on videodisc one to the turning sequence on videodisc two. If the student did not execute the turn, it would keep playing videodisc one through the intersection at which point the instructor's voice would say, "You should have turned there." An even more realistic simulator could be created by using multiple cameras and videodiscs, a spherical projection television screen, and computer-controlled image processing to provide zoom, tilt, and pan capabilities. Admittedly, this type of simulator would be quite expensive to construct, but the fact that the possibility *exists* suggests exciting options for future simulators. Instead of using computer-generated graphics to represent real-world scenes, simulator designers will be able to select video images of the real world, and modify them to suit the situation.

Another type of simulation that has especially attractive applications in education is the simulation game. In this type of program, the student is expected to cope with a simulated situation, and his or her performance is compared to an ideal performance by invoking a scoring rule. Whether a simulation is a game depends on the player; when the National Aeronautics and Space Administration (NASA) built their lunar lander simulator, they did not think of it as a game. But today, almost any programmable calculator can run a simplified lunar lander simulation as an entertainment. For a physics student, such a situation is both a game ("How close can I come to a perfect landing?") and a lesson in Newtonian mechanics.

We believe that simulation games can be especially effective in teaching topics that require interaction between humans, such as the teaching of foreign languages. We are developing a program that simulates a visit to a Mexican village. It begins with a panoramic view of the central plaza of the town. From one corner of the plaza, a man is seen approaching the camera. When he arrives at a conversational distance, he asks (in Spanish), "You're an American tourist, aren't you?" and his image freezes. If the student indicates that the statement was understood, the computer controlling the videodisc program writes a number of possible answers to the statement, in English, on the control screen. (If the statement was not understood, the scene is repeated.) The student is required to pick an answer, translate it into Spanish, and speak it into a microphone that is connected to a voice-actuated tape recorder. To the computer, the student just indicates which answer he or she proposes to give. When the answer has been given in Spanish, the student presses a button and sees a surrogate student giving the same answer in Spanish to the inquisitive gentleman. The native then replies with an explanation or another question, and the dialogue continues. At the end of the session, the audiotape, with all of the student's voice productions, can be reviewed by an instructor for correct pronunciation. The "game" aspect of

this simulation is in exploring an unknown (and unpredict-
able) village, and coping with unexpected developments. The
possible scenarios include a visit to the market, bargaining to
purchase a leather briefcase, a taxi ride to the bullfights, a
meal in the best restaurant in town, or a night at a disco with
a Mariachi band. The program has just one starting point, but
eight ending points, so the student is motivated to "explore"
the village, starting each time from the central plaza and
opting for different routes through the village. Because the
Spanish language makes more gender distinctions than
English, our program will assume that the student is male on
one side of the disc and female on the other side. Naturally,
the sex of the surrogate student will match the assumption,
so that the simulation will be equally realistic for students of
both sexes.

Another language application is the development of
annotated foreign films. For example, we have taken a classic
Mexican film, MACARIO, and added an English language
soundtrack. We only wanted to use one side of a videodisc
for this project, so we selected what we thought were the 27
most important minutes of the dialogue, and added about
130 still-frame sequences to illustrate the remaining portions
of the program. This material was transferred from 35mm
film to videodisc. The rest of the audio tracks (English and
Spanish) were further edited and dubbed to an audiocassette.
To present the movie, we connect our videodisc player and
an audiocassette deck to a small computer. The show begins
when the computer instructs the videodisc player to put up a
series of still frames for the titles and credits, while the
audiocassette player plays the theme music. After the credits
have rolled by, the computer shows a motion sequence from
the videodisc. After that, some more still frames from the
videodisc are displayed, accompanied by dialogue from the
cassette. A special "stop" button is wired to the computer so
that the student can press it and stop the show whenever he

or she has a question, or whenever he or she misses the meaning of the Spanish dialogue. Whenever the show is stopped, the computer displays a set of six control options on its console, and also displays a variable number (usually seven to 12) of topical questions that the student might have about the interrupted scene. Figure 16 shows a diagram of this overall scheme. We have stored 29 different question menus in the computer, so when the student presses the stop button, the computer must figure out which menu is appropriate to this section of the film, retrieve it, and display it. The topical questions on the menus refer to a wide range of aspects of the film: the symbolism of a felled tree, or the allegorical nature of some of the characters, or the style of dress, or some history about the Spanish Inquisition. The six control options are the same for all menus. These options allow the student to continue from the point where the program stopped, to go back to the beginning of the scene, to return a second time and hear the dialogue in English, to go back to the previous scene, or to end the program. The annotated movie is one example of existing linear material being refitted for use with interactive videodiscs.

The annotated movie technique is equally applicable in other content areas. Andrew Lippman at MIT has developed a "personalized" movie on bicycle maintenance that uses a similar technique. It allows the user to access the disc either for reference purposes or as a tutorial device. It will display an exploded view drawing, call out the nomenclature, or show the viewer the entire step-by-step process for repacking a wheel bearing.

Another, more global, example of a "refit" is the building of a videodisc-based information system nicknamed "Data-land." Richard A. Bolt of MIT has developed such a system, formally known as the Spatial Data-Management System. Figure 17 cannot begin to do justice to the elaborate apparatus in the MIT Media Room where the SDMS is being

Figure 16

Branching Options for Interactive Videodisc "MACARIO"

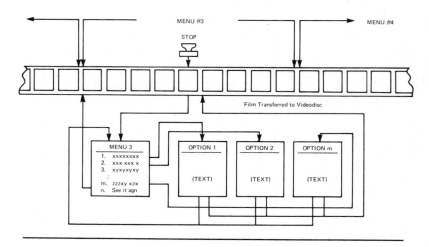

Figure 17

MIT "Media Room," with Rear-Projection Video,
Touch-Sensitive Video Monitors, and Octophonic Sound

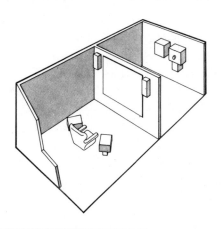

implemented. In addition to computers and videodiscs, there is a huge rear-projection screen, two color monitors with touch-sensitive screens, an electronic writing and drawing tablet, octophonic sound, and a large easychair with "joy-stick" and touch-sensitive controls built into the armrests. The system gives the occupant of the armchair a sense of movement and of direction, as he or she peruses the various items of information stored in "Dataland." The importance of this application is not in the esoteric hardware but in the use of realistic visual images to represent the position of an observer in a pseudo-spatial structure. Without the image retrieval system, Dataland would be just another messy office.

You could develop your own "Spatial Data-Management System" if you were to take all of your paraphernalia: your slides, movies, audiocassettes, reports, books, calendars, computer printouts, even your telephone and your pocket calculator, and lay them all out on a nice grassy meadow. Now, climb into the bucket of a "cherry picker" hoist and pull the lever to go up, up, up, until you have a panoramic view of the entire domain. Your very own "Dataland"! To access a particular item, you position the cherry picker's arm in the X-Y planes and then zoom in (the Z plane) by lowering the bucket. Although the cherry picker can move in three dimensions, the paraphernalia is located in two dimensions, and must stay where it is placed. The cherry picker's third dimension is comparable to the magnification setting on a microscope. Future versions of MIT's Dataland will overcome these limitations, allowing the viewer to reorganize information with multidimensional attributes.

Judging by these initial applications, videodiscs will not be restricted to one content area, nor to one instructional method, nor to one method of distribution. The wide variety of applications should accelerate the spread of this technology to every segment of the educational community. Because videodiscs offer previously unavailable capabilities as well as improvements in reliability, durability, and economy, they will prosper by the development of totally new applications—and not just by displacing existing audiovisual equipment.

4.

Videodisc Economics

By "economics," we mean a relative type of economics; a comparison of different alternatives for the production and delivery of mediated instruction. We will consider four instructional situations:

(1) the presentation of a linear (i.e., conventional) "motion picture" program;

(2) the presentation of a collection of individual still frames, to be shown in a teacher-selected, arbitrary sequence;

(3) a mixed-mode presentation combining motion picture and still-frame materials; and

(4) an interactive videodisc compared to computer-assisted instruction (CAI).

Before we discuss these situations in detail, a few points are in order. Except in the simplest case of direct transfer from pre-existing material to videodisc, videodisc technology, or more correctly the use of videodisc as a system component, affects not only the design and cost of the delivery system, but also the instructional design and production systems. This is so because the features provided by the videodisc allow instructional developers to use visual materials in different ways, qualitatively as well as quantitatively. Similarly, the economic comparisons are not just a matter of looking at price tags and quantity discounts. These costs of acquisition are only the tip of the iceberg. The really important cost is the cost of ownership, which includes acquisition costs as well as durability of the product (the expected length of service) and the cost of making repairs when they are needed. Another important point is that media systems have two components: hardware (the player or projector) and software (the material containing images, sound, etc.). Meaningful comparisons can only be made when both components are evaluated as a single package.

For our first situation, suppose that we have a one-hour video program that we wish to distribute. Which medium will provide the lowest per-copy cost? The answer is: it depends very much on the number of copies that will be distributed. Table 4 gives the per-copy costs for 16mm motion picture film, 3/4-inch videocassettes, and optical videodiscs. We see that the initial costs for film and for videodiscs are many times higher than the one-copy costs for videocassettes, but as the number of copies increases, the cost functions cross. Figure 18 shows what happens for large quantities. These are the same data given in Table 4, plotted on logarithmic scales. The Figure shows that the cost of 139 videodiscs is the same as the cost of 139 cassettes. So we see that the price quoted for a single copy does not tell the whole story; it is the number of copies you want that really makes the decision.

These curves demonstrate another important feature of videodiscs: they provide protection against pirating—the illegal manufacture of bootleg copies. It is not that the disc self-destructs when you attempt to make a videotape copy of it, nor will the marketplace for videodiscs be any easier to control than the current market for videocassettes. The protection is economic protection; when large quantities of videodiscs are produced, it is cheaper to buy another copy of the videodisc than it is to buy blank videocassettes and spend the time copying the contents of the disc. For this to be true of materials distributed on videocassettes, the producer must

Figure 18

---

*Per-Copy Media Duplication Costs for
One-Hour Program, Originating on Videotape*

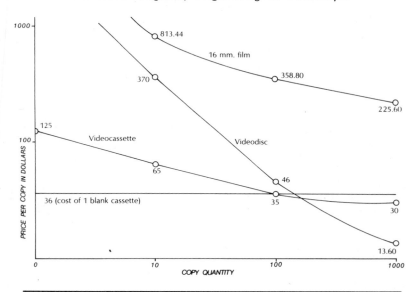

Table 4

Per-Copy Media Costs for a One-Hour Program

Medium	Copy Quantity			
	1	10	100	1,000
16mm Color Film (includes inter-negative, etc.)	$4,875	813	359	226
3/4-inch Videocassettes	125	65	35	30
Videodiscs	3,610	370	46	14

drastically limit marketing and program production costs so that he or she can sell cassettes for no more than the cost of making a single copy. Because videocassettes have a relatively flat cost-quantity function, this is virtually impossible. So the producer must sell the cassette for much more than the blank cassette costs and be resigned to the fact that each cassette sold will probably be copied several times, thereby reducing the size of the market for additional copies. With videodiscs, the producer is in a much better position to recoup the investment and retain the market: he or she can charge almost three times the cost of the disc copy before exceeding the cost of a single blank cassette. This characteristic of videodiscs should make them a much more attractive distribution medium for producers of high-quality, high-cost programming. Unfortunately, the future is a bit clouded due to the rapid growth of low-cost, half-inch video formats (Betamax and VHS). For these formats, blank tapes cost between $2.40 and $7.25 per hour, depending on the image quality desired. We believe that this threat is strong motivation for videodisc manufacturers to reduce media costs as rapidly as the developing technology will allow.

Now that the media costs have been examined, we need to look at the costs associated with a reasonably complete instructional system. To do this, we will expand on the model developed by Carter and Walker (1969) for an earlier cost study of instructional television and computer-assisted instruction:

> For the purposes of this study, the basic school unit is assumed to be a theoretical district with 100,000 students in grades one through 12. Each school district has 152 school centers, comprising 76 elementary schools and 76 secondary schools. Each school has 24 classrooms, and there is a total of 3,648 classrooms in the school system. The elementary schools have 30 students per classroom and 720 students per school, while the secondary schools have 25 students per classroom and 600 students per school. The number, class size, and enrollments of the theoretical

district's schools were established for statistical and computational purposes only.

Now, suppose that we want to provide one hour of programming per student per day for 12 grades for 150 school days. This would require 1,800 lessons for the school year. We will consider two types of delivery systems in this situation. The first are network systems, implying closed-circuit television, and using either videotape players or videodisc players or film chains at the point of transmission. The second are local "roll-around" systems located in each school building. We will have six roll-around systems in each building, each one averaging four hours a day of use. For the network system, we will assume that the classrooms are wired and that there are 12 portable television monitors for each school. The model for these configurations is illustrated in Figures 19a and 19b.

Table 5 lists the component costs, and Table 6 shows the cost analysis for these alternatives. The cost of the initial equipment acquisition is given in the first column, and the second column is the cost of acquiring media. In the case of the network systems, two complete copies of all of the lessons are purchased for the head end. In the case of the local systems, two copies of the elementary lessons or three copies of the secondary lessons are available at each school. The fourth column, annual operating costs, reflects the cost of staffing and administering a central transmission facility. The operating costs for the local systems are absorbed by the personnel at the individual schools. The annual maintenance costs are estimated at five percent of the acquisition cost for electronic components, and 12 percent for mechanical ones. The annual equipment replacement costs are based on amortization figures for each component of the system under study. For example, a videotape player is amortized in three years, so one-third of the replacement costs is budgeted each year. The last column gives the ten-year total, which is the

Figure 19a

Network Configuration for
Hypothetical School District

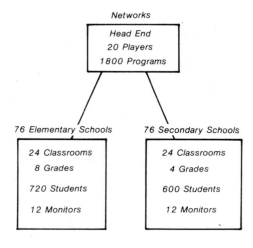

Networks

Head End
20 Players
1800 Programs

76 Elementary Schools   76 Secondary Schools

24 Classrooms   24 Classrooms
8 Grades   4 Grades
720 Students   600 Students
12 Monitors   12 Monitors

Figure 19b

Local Distribution Configuration
for Hypothetical School District

Local Systems

76 Elementary Schools   76 Secondary Schools

24 Classrooms   24 Classrooms
1200 Programs   600 Programs
6 Players   6 Players
12 Monitors   12 Monitors
or   or
6 Projectors   6 Projectors
24 Screens   24 Screens

Table 5

Cost Estimates Used in Delivery System Example

Component	Purchase Cost	Useful Life
16mm Projector	$ 773.	3 years
Screen	77.	2
Color TV Receiver	650.	5
3/4" VTR	1,875.	3
Videodisc Player	2,000.	5
Film Chain	15,000.	4
Microwave Receiver	3,000.	10
Transmitter and Studio	300,000.	10
16mm Film	See Table 4.	50 plays
3/4" Videotape Cassette	See Table 4.	150 plays
Videodisc	See Table 4.	Unlimited

Table 6

Ten-Year Costs (in Thousands of Dollars) for Alternative Delivery Systems

Type of System	Acquisition			Average Annual Costs					10 yr. Total
	Equipment	Media	Total	Operating	Maintenance	Equipment	Media	Total	
Network									
CCTV w/Film Chain	2,556	1,173	3,729	90	133	388	70	681	10,539
CCTV w/VTR	2,344	288	2,632	33	118	325	6	482	7,452
CCTV w/Videodisc	2,346	6,516	8,862	33	117	321	0	471	13,572
Self-Contained Local									
16mm Film (from video)	986	111,720	112,706	--	118	375	3,830	4,323	155,936
16mm Film (from negative)	986	92,370	93,356	--	118	375	3,159	3,652	129,875
3/4" Videotape Cassette	2,896	11,172	14,068	--	179	807	128	1,114	25,208
Videodisc	3,010	9,672	12,682	--	150	602	0	752	20,202

acquisition cost plus ten times the annual costs. In this analysis, the total cost of the network systems is much less than any of the local in-school systems. In the network application, videodisc is not cost-effective. The reason for this is seen in the media acquisition column. Because so few copies of each lesson are purchased when all of the lessons are stored centrally, videotape is a much more economical format than videodisc. By contrast, in the local systems, hundreds of copies of each program must be made, and the videodisc system acquits itself very well. The ten-year costs for a local videodisc system are 20 percent less than the costs for 3/4" videotape. The videotape, in turn, is a real bargain compared to 16mm films. In the 16mm local systems, the low hardware acquisition costs are washed out by the expensive media costs. The contrast between film and videodisc is especially strong in the annual media cost column. The small difference between the two film systems demonstrates that the cost of transferring from videotape to film is overshadowed by the cost of making release prints.

This example was chosen to demonstrate the effect of life-cycle costs, and not to show off videodiscs. To do the latter, we would have chosen a situation with thousands of copies of each program, and each program would have been played over and over, to demonstrate the value of a medium that does not wear out.

Now, let's look at an entirely different situation: a situation where a very large mediabase of still visuals is to be reproduced. Table 7 shows the costs that would be incurred if the mediabase were to be reproduced as 35mm slides, 35mm filmstrips, microfiche, or videodisc. To make the numbers as impressive as possible, we have chosen the maximum capacity of a double-sided disc. In the admittedly extreme case of a thousand copies of this large number of images, videodisc has a tremendous price advantage over 35mm

Table 7

Per-Frame Costs, in Dollars,
for Copies of a Large
Set of Still Visuals (108,000)

Medium	Number of Copies			
	1	10	100	1,000
35mm color slides	0.33	0.26	0.20	0.12
35mm color filmstrips	0.16	0.03	0.01	0.01
Microfiche, color	0.20	0.03	0.01	0.01
Videodisc	0.04	0.004	0.0006	0.00002

slides—more than one thousand to one. But this is one situation where making even a *single* disc would be worthwhile. The "break-even" point between 35mm slides and videodisc comes at 5,477 slides. In theory, for slide collections larger than this, videodisc, even just a single videodisc, is less expensive. (Of course, we are ignoring the fact that videodisc manufacturers usually insist on replicating a minimum of 50 discs.)

The third situation is a mixture of the first two; still frames mixed in with motion sequences. This is the arrangement which we have used in our "MACARIO" annotated movie, and the situation which we believe will be most prevalent when videodiscs are used with computer-based instruction. The situation is economically interesting because the cost of preparing still frames and the cost of preparing motion sequences are counter-balanced by the amount of time which students spend on the material. Figure 20, updated from Bennion and Schneider (1975), shows that in terms of the cost of instruction per hour, the function is relatively flat over a wide range of mixtures of still frames and motion sequences. The Figure also makes the point that the easiest way to achieve low-cost instruction with video-discs is by mass distribution of the material. Building a large-scale educational market has never been easy, but it is certainly possible, as book publishers have demonstrated for many years.

The fourth situation, interactive videodisc versus CAI, contains all of the preceding cost considerations and several new unknowns. Interactive videodisc systems are still in developmental stages, but we suspect that a computer-based system with a small "floppy disc" mass memory could be marketed for about $5,000. Depending on the requirements of the application, alternatives could range from a videotape-based responder system (about $3,250) to full-color high-resolution computer graphics systems costing $10,000 to $40,000. Another highly variable factor is the cost of instructional development; in some cases where the content is fairly abstract, videodiscs might cost the same as computer programs. In situations requiring a great deal of realism, computer graphics could be several orders of magnitude more expensive. In the long run, we expect the dichotomy between videodisc systems and computer graphic systems to blur, and an amalgam of the two will emerge, with videodiscs providing basic, permanent information, and computer-generated graphic overlays providing details that may vary from student to student.

A few words should be said about the relative cost trends for various media. In the last few years, the cost of paper has shown a steady and sizable increase. More recently, rising silver prices have driven up film costs by 30 percent to 50 percent. Magnetic tape has not been as volatile as paper and

Figure 20

Cost Per Hour of Instructional Material
as a Function of the Proportion of the Videodisc
Containing Still Frames (Shown for Several Copy Quantities)

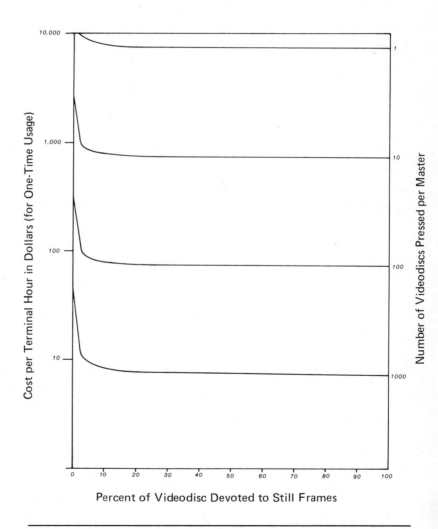

Percent of Videodisc Devoted to Still Frames

film, but it has also been increasing. The cost improvements offered by half-inch tape formats have come from improvements in the players, not in the tape. (Further improvements may come from metallic tapes and from amorphous metals, but they will command higher prices.) In the meantime, videodisc replication techniques have been improving fairly rapidly, and the cost of discs has been *decreasing*. Competitive mastering and replication services are just tooling up. As a result, the relative cost advantage of videodiscs is very likely to increase during the coming decade. In fact, if these trends continue, *videodisc* may be the only medium we can *afford* by the end of this decade.

5.

How Are Videodiscs Made?

Although it is possible to master a videodisc directly using live, real-time action observed by a video camera, this process is never used due to the need to edit programs before mastering, and due to the elaborate clean-room environment needed for the mastering process. Other media (videotape and film) are used to store and edit the motion and audio sequences prior to mastering. These media can be almost any format (35, 16, or 8mm film; 3/4, one, or two-inch videotape). However, the quality of the videodisc cannot be better than that of the original source. Therefore, it is advisable to use broadcast-quality recording systems and to interpose as few generations (copies) as possible between the original footage and the videodisc master.

What follows is a description of the procedures used by DiscoVision Associates (DVA) to master and replicate reflective videodiscs. (Mastering means transferring the program to a glass master disc; replication means making the copies.) We understand that a virtually identical process is used by Philips in the Netherlands, and that the Thomson-CSF process is the same for mastering, but differs considerably in replication. A number of radically different replication processes have been considered in the past, and a number of new ones are being developed, so do not be surprised if a different replication process is used when you are ready to produce your own discs. (For example, 3M Corporation has announced that it will offer replication services for Thomson discs starting in the fourth quarter of 1980, and will do the same for reflective discs by the first part of 1981. They plan to use a casting process, instead of injection molding, and to make a composite disc, using one type of plastic for the body of the disc and another for the micropits.)

Transfer

Unless you walk in with a two-inch helical-format videotape, the first thing that DVA does is to transfer your material to that format, and add the videodisc frame numbers at the same time. If your material is film, they will use a Rank-Cintel flying-spot scanner to convert the film frames to video frames. If your film has been shot at 24 frames per second, the standard speed for sound films, the equipment will have to add an extra video frame for every four film frames so that the transferred material will conform to the television standard of 30 frames per second. The extra frame is made by taking information from two consecutive film frames and creating a kind of "double exposure" video frame. This frame is completely unnoticeable at normal viewing speeds, but in slow-motion and freeze-frame modes it would be very distracting. To keep the player from freezing on these composite frames, the frame-numbering hardware does not assign them a frame number, and the player is built so that it will not freeze on an unnumbered frame. So the highest frame number on a half-hour disc made from a film source will be 43,200, not 54,000, although the disc actually has 54,000 "spaces" available.

Mastering

Video images and sound signals are merged into one composite signal for mastering videodiscs. This composite signal modulates the energy source used to create the information pattern on the master videodisc. There are three methods currently used to create master discs: they can be recorded by (1) laser techniques (optical discs), (2) modulating an electron beam (RCA), or (3) using a mechanical cutting process similar to that used to generate audiodisc masters (TED).

The DVA mastering process begins with the preparation of a circular glass plate about 1/4-inch in thickness and 14 inches in diameter. The surface of the glass plate is very carefully ground, using extremely fine abrasives to remove all of the surface marks or pits. It is then polished to form a very smooth, optically flat surface. This surface is coated with a positive photo-resistant material similar to that used to make printed circuit boards. The glass master disc is then placed onto a motor-driven spindle that rotates at 1,800 rpm for CAV discs and a gradually decreasing speed for CLV discs.

The mastering equipment includes the spindle and an optical bench set-up to focus the laser beam onto the rotating master disc (see Figure 21). The program source material frequency-modulates an eight Megahertz carrier signal, and it in turn modulates a blue (argon gas) laser beam. Modulation of the light is done by intermittently blocking the beam with a very high-speed light switch. Specifically, the beam is blocked during one-half of each cycle (see Figure 22). During the other half cycle, the laser beam is allowed to pass, thus exposing the photo-resistant material on the master disc. A lead screw drive moves the beam slowly across the face of the rotating disc, forming a spiral pattern, or track. Each revolution of the track is separated by only 65 millionths of an inch.

After the photo-resistant material on the glass master has been exposed by the recording laser beam, the master disc is developed, which removes the exposed resistant material to form microscopic three-dimensional pits. This surface is then metalized with an evaporated metal coating. Additional

Figure 21

Mastering Lathe for Reflective Videodiscs

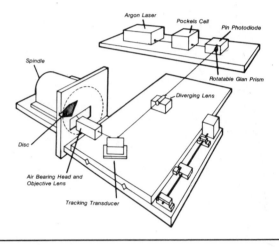

Figure 22

Relationships Between the Composite Television Signal,
the Switched Laser Beam, and the Resulting Disc

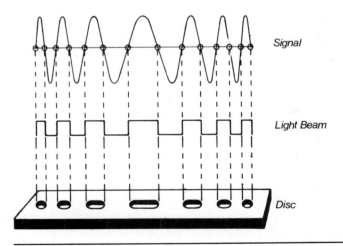

processing with conventional electroplating techniques produces a nickel "mother" from which a submaster is made. The final product of this process is a "stamper," which is essentially a mirror image of the original photo-resistant surface.

Replication

The stamper is used to produce replicas. Thousands of replicas can be made from multiple submasters and stampers. The DVA method of replication is injection molding; the stamper is placed on one side of a special injection molding press. When the two halves of the mold are pressed together, a cavity is formed, and molten acrylic plastic is injected. The mold is then cooled. After the plastic has solidified, the mold is opened and the plastic is removed.

Another method of replication uses an ultra-violet stabilized polymer. With this method, the "stamper" is coated with a liquid polymer, which is then exposed to a strong ultra-violet light. Upon exposure, the liquid polymer reacts, and it is transformed to rigid plastic. Either process produces a one-sided videodisc. The side containing the micropits of this clear plastic disc is then coated with a thin reflective metallic layer. Two of these one-sided discs are bonded together, back to back, to form the finished videodisc.

Slightly different procedures are used in replicating the transmissive videodisc. The stamper is used to emboss a clear polyvinyl chloride (PVC) disc. No reflective layer or scuffcoat is applied, and the disc must be protected from direct handling and from dust.

Mastering Mechanically-Read Discs

The information on the TED master disc is generated by using the same mechanical cutting process that is used for producing audio records. However, instead of allowing the cutting needle to move sideways, as is done for audio records, the needle is forced to move only in a vertical direction (perpendicular to the surface of the disc). The reason for using a vertical movement of the cutting needle becomes apparent when we see that the grooves on the TED disc are separated by only 3.5 micrometers, whereas grooves on an audio record are separated by a 50-times greater distance. These variations in depth are then transferred to the replicated discs using audio record-stamping techniques. The TED master is not recorded in real time; the cutting lathe turns at 45 rpm or less, and the playback spindle turns at 1,800 rpm. As a result, it takes six hours and 40 minutes to master a ten-minute disc. For this reason, only film is used for source material because it can be advanced very slowly, a frame at a time.

Once the master has been cut, replicas are made by stamping the information on thin (and therefore flexible) discs of polyvinyl chloride (PVC) plastic.

RCA SelectaVision videodiscs are mastered by using an electron beam process. The master disc has a copper substrate base (see Figure 23) that is grooved in a spiral pattern. An electron-sensitive material is coated over these grooves to form an undulating surface. The electron beam is directed from an electron microscope through a series of "lenses" to provide a finely focused beam of electrons at the surface of the master disc. This beam of electrons is turned on and off to provide the desired exposure.

A turntable moves the master disc under the electron beam in a spiral pattern to expose the disc. The rotation is controlled by a hydraulic turbine and an optical tachometer. Special servo circuits maintain the electron beam on track.

After exposure and development, the relief pattern on the master disc is transferred to submasters and stampers with the same methods used for audio records. The replicated discs have a metallic surface applied and are then coated with a styrene dielectric coat and a final coat of silicone oil, which

Figure 23

Cross-section of RCA Mastering Disc

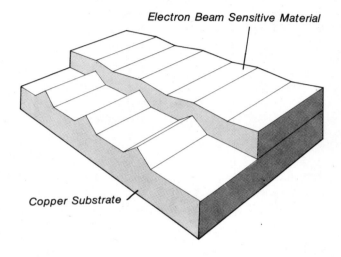

Electron Beam Sensitive Material

Copper Substrate

acts as a lubricant to increase the life of both the record and the stylus.

Historically, the electron beam recording system has not had enough energy to expose the photo-resistant material on the disc at real-time recording speeds. Most of the laboratory recordings have utilized a 20-times slower recording speed. Increases in both electron beam energy and sensitivity of the photo-resistant material may permit real-time recording techniques to be used eventually. In the meantime, film will be the only acceptable source format.

The JVC videodisc mastering system uses a laser beam to expose a photo-resistant material coated to a glass master disc. The microscopic pits are arranged with their long axis at right angles to the track. The master disc rotates at 900 rpm to allow two video frames per revolution. Separate tracking signals are also created during mastering. A metal stamper is made from the glass master disc after it has been processed to form the pits. Conventional audiodisc processes are employed to produce videodiscs from the stamper.

For the educational user, the mastering technique is not as important as the cost and durability of the finished product. The costs of mastering should be roughly comparable for most of these techniques, because they are just variants of the same basic process. The big differences are in the quality of the replicas and their durability in the hands of typical users. We expect to see a continuous trickle of small improvements in both of these areas over the next few years.

6.

Industrial/Educational Videodisc Players

"Industrial" model videodisc players, which for the purpose of this book we have dubbed industrial/educational players, are to the home entertainment players as studio monitors are to home television sets; they are designed to run all day, every day, and they have additional control capabilities that give the user (and the user's computer system) maximum flexibility in deciding what to look at next.

The two industrial/educational model players, the Disco-Vision PR7820 and the Thomson-CSF TTV3620 (Figures 13 and 10, respectively), are capable of searching out a particular frame and of being interfaced to an external computer. In both cases, these extra features are provided by installing a microprocessor to control all of the player functions. The PR7820 uses a Fairchild microprocessor, while the TTV3620 uses a Motorola chip. From this point on, the two players diverge radically.

The DVA PR7820 Videodisc Player

The PR7820 player comes with a remote-control unit (see Figure 24) that can be used in a cradle on top of the machine, or it can be hand-held. It communicates with the player by transmitting infra-red signals. The transmitters are located in the top end of the unit, and the receiver is behind

Figure 24

DiscoVision Associates Model RU-8
Remote Control Unit
(for use with the DVA PR7820 player)

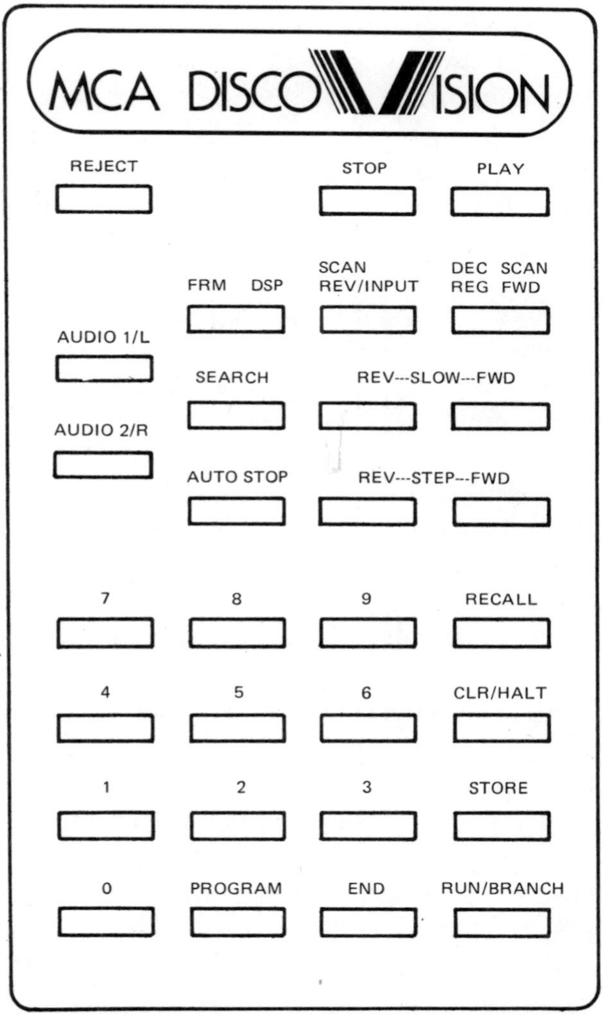

MCA DISCOVISION

REJECT		STOP	PLAY

FRM	DSP	SCAN REV/INPUT	DEC SCAN REG FWD

AUDIO 1/L

	SEARCH	REV---SLOW---FWD	

AUDIO 2/R

	AUTO STOP	REV---STEP---FWD	

7	8	9	RECALL

4	5	6	CLR/HALT

1	2	3	STORE

0	PROGRAM	END	RUN/BRANCH

a one-inch diameter black disc to the right of the push-buttons on the control panel of the player.

The pushbuttons on the remote unit duplicate most of the front-panel controls and provide programming controls as well. Programming the player means putting the machine in program mode and then entering a string of numbers and commands into the machine's memory. Before we describe the commands, we need to make some distinctions among the various things that get numbered in a videodisc program.

Different Things That Get Numbered

There are three types of numbers you should know. These are frame numbers, register numbers, and program step numbers.

Frame Numbers: Every accessible picture or frame on the disc is numbered. These numbers are important for locating any specific place on the disc, and they must be used to make programming possible. If you push "FRM DSP" (see Figure 24, row 2, column 2), the frame number of the frame being displayed will appear in the upper left-hand part of the screen. Push it again and the number is removed. Frame numbers start at zero and can go as high as 54,000.

Register Numbers: Register numbers range from 0 to 511. The registers are located in the machine's memory, and are used to store specific frame numbers for quick recall. To load the registers, just key in the number of the register desired, then push "RECALL" (see Figure 24, row 5, column 4). The numbers displayed on the screen show the register number and the frame number that are stored in that register. If you wish to store a different number in that register, you key in the number of the frame desired, then push the "STORE" (see Figure 24, row 7, column 4) button. The number will be stored, and the contents of the next sequential register will be displayed. This is very handy when a sequence of registers is being loaded. Similarly, pressing "RECALL" repeatedly will let you review the contents of a series of registers.

The registers have several uses. If certain pictures or frames are to be selected from the rest of the disc, the desired frame numbers can be loaded into any of the registers (one per register). Suppose you want to display the frame whose number is stored in register 2; you push "2," "RECALL," then "SEARCH" (see Figure 24, row 3, column 2). (SEARCH is the command used to locate a specific frame on the disc.) The machine will then search out and display the frame whose number is loaded in that register.

Program Step Numbers: When using the program mode, each key-press in the program is automatically numbered. Program step numbers range from "0" to "1023." If you wish to check to see what has been placed on any program step, just key in the number of the program step desired, then push PROGRAM (see Figure 24, row 8, column 2). The display will show on the screen, the top line indicating the program step number keyed in, and the bottom line the entry. Each time the PROGRAM button is keyed, the next step will be displayed. To leave the program mode, the END (see Figure 24, row 8, column 3) button is pressed.

Registers and program steps share the same memory space. They start at opposite ends of memory. Each register uses the space of two program steps. Register "0" occupies the same space as steps "1022" and "1023"; register "1" corresponds to steps 1020 and 1021. Program steps "0" and "1" correspond to register "511," while steps "2" and "3" correspond to register "510."

Programming

Just to give a feel for what it is like to program a videodisc, let's run through a small example:

Suppose we start our program at frame number 3400, play to frame number 4000, and then stop. First push "0," then PROGRAM. You are now in the program mode, starting at program step zero. Next, key in: "3400," "SEARCH" (SRC),

"4000 AUTO STOP" (ATP), then "HALT" (HLT), and "END" (END). The halt used in this manner stops the program from executing any more program steps. The END button terminates the programming mode.

Editing Programs: Suppose you changed your mind and decided to make the sample program above stop at frame 4500 instead of 4000. Instead of rekeying the entire program, you can edit the 0 after the 4, and change it to a 5. To do this, you have to locate the program step that holds that 0. This can be done by stepping through the program by repeatedly pressing the PGM key until you arrive, or by counting the number of steps on your programming form, counting one step for each digit and one step for each command. Our program starts at step 0, so the 0 you want to change is located in step 6. Key in: "6 PGM, 5, END" and the change is complete. If you stepped through the program, stop when you get to step 6, key in: "5, END," and you are done.

Run Mode: To run the program, just push the "0" and "RUN" buttons. If the program starts at a program step other than 0, key in the starting step in place of 0. The program will run until it encounters a HALT command, or you push the CLR/HALT button. If the RUN command is not preceded by a number, 0 is assumed.

Programming Commands

Each command is explained in this section. They are organized (more or less) in order of increasing complexity and decreasing frequency of usage.

SEARCH: This command is used to position the disc to a specific frame. The desired frame may be numbered either higher or lower than the current frame.

AUTO STOP: This command lets you set a desired frame number and have the machine play to that point and stop. If the frame number you specify is less than the current frame, AUTO STOP becomes equivalent to SEARCH.

WAIT: To create a pause in the program, you must use the STOP button. The length of the pause in seconds must be multiplied by ten. This number is then keyed in, followed by "STOP." (In program mode, the STOP key displays WAIT on the screen.)

SLOW MOTION: This may be put in a program by keying in the frame number at which slow motion is to stop, followed by SLOW FWD or SLOW REV. We will give these as "SLF" or "SLR." This should be followed by the next step you wish in your program.

AUDIO: Audio channels may be changed or turned off completely in a program by keying AUDIO 1 or AUDIO 2 following a stop in action. It must be followed by another command which would resume action. To turn the audio "off," key in a "0," then AUDIO 1 or AUDIO 2. To turn the audio "on," use a "1" just prior to keying AUDIO. If the audio commands are not preceded by a number, they will just reverse the existing condition. If the channel is on, it will go off, and if it is off, it will go on.

The player is wired so that the left channel, channel 1, will automatically switch between the two soundtracks. If you are listening to the channel 1 output and you turn off channel 1 with channel 2 on, you will hear channel 2 on the channel 1 circuit. When channel 1 is turned on again, you will hear only channel 1.

FRAME DISPLAY (FRM DSP): This can be turned on or off during a program in the same manner as AUDIO. Unless FRM DSP is preceded by "0" (for "off") or "1" (for "on"), it will simply reverse the existing condition; if absent, the frame number will appear; if present, it will disappear.

HALT (CLR/HALT): This command stops execution of the program (removes machine from run mode). The show does not necessarily stop; the player continues to do whatever it was doing when the HALT (HLT) instruction was encountered. In direct control mode, this button clears the register display from the screen.

BRANCH (RUN/BRANCH): If you wish a program to repeat itself indefinitely, i.e., "loop," then at the end of the program, just before the HLT, you can key in "0 BRANCH (BRN)." Your program will now run continuously until you stop it by pushing "HALT." The number keyed in preceding BRANCH should be the program step number where your program began, if it did not begin at "0."

Of course, you can make a smaller loop out of just the last portion of your program; the BRANCH command can go to any program step. If no program step precedes the BRANCH command, the program branches to step 0.

INPUT (SCAN REV/INPUT): INPUT, used in connection with BRANCH, gives you the option of having several programs and choosing between them. For instance, in a multiple-choice test item, a student may be asked to press button 0, 1, or 2, corresponding to his or her selection of an answer to a question. Each selection would be programmed to explain a given topic or clear up a particular misconception. At the end of each branch of the program, the program would return to the starting point to await another selection, or go on to the next question.

DECREMENT REGISTER (DEC REG/SCAN FWD): This command allows a program to repeat a loop a predetermined number of times, and then either terminate or continue with more programmed material. This type of repetition can be useful when teaching new perceptual-motor skills. An instructor may wish to have a certain learning task repeated several times before moving on to other areas. A language teacher may wish to have some material repeated several times in a foreign language, and then the same thing repeated in English.

Before entering the DEC REG loop for the first time, a register must be selected and the number of passes through the loop must be loaded into it. The loading occurs in the regular way, using the STORE command. Next, the program steps that will be in the loop are entered into the program memory. At the end of the loop, the DEC REG command is used to decrease the register contents by one. Following this command is the program step number where the loop begins, followed in turn by a BRN command. Every time the DEC REG command is encountered, it decrements the recalled register and then compares the new value to zero. If the value is greater than zero, the program steps immediately following the DEC REG command are executed. If the value is equal to zero, the processor skips steps until it finds a BRN command, and then resumes execution with the first step after the BRN. If you want to use the same loop again, be sure to reload the countdown register before reentering.

Multiple Programs. You can put in as many programs as will fit in the player's memory, starting your programs at different program step numbers and ending each with a HLT. To RUN a program that does not start at program step zero, prefix the RUN command with the starting step number.

Retaining Programs in Memory

Turning off the machine's power does not destroy the contents of memory. Even if the power cord is unplugged, the memory will hold its contents until the next day. Memory contents are modified by writing new steps over the old ones, or playing a disc with a pre-recorded program dump.

Thomson-CSF TTV3620 Videodisc Player

This player's remote-control unit is shown in Figure 25. It has only half as many keys as the PR7820 because it uses a different command structure, and it does not store programs. In this section, we will describe very briefly the way the player works when it "stands alone," reserving the computer-connection features for the next chapter.

Once the disc is loaded, and the "Local-Ext." switch (Figure

Figure 25

Thomson-CSF TTV3620 Remote Control Unit

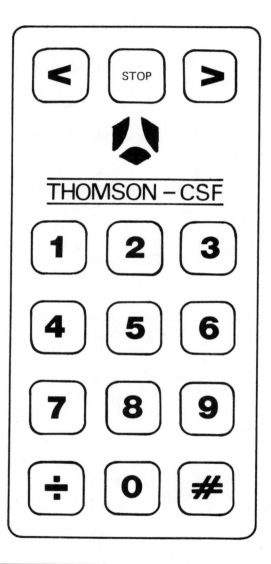

10) is in the "Local" position, you start by setting the read-out speed. The Thomson player treats speed as a continuum in the sense that the normal 30-frame advances per second is treated as just another speed. In another sense, the speeds are quite discrete; there are nine selectable speeds, from 60-frame advances per second to one-frame advance every 4.27 seconds; a ratio of 256:1. The double-time speed, 60 fps, is obtained by pressing the "2" button. All of the other speeds are selected by pressing "9," followed by a digit from "0" to "7": "0" means normal, "1" means half normal, "2" means one-fourth normal, and so forth; successive halvings until "7," which equals 1/128 of normal.

The other functions of the player are essentially those of the Pioneer VP-1000 unit. All of the "standard" mode (i.e., stand-alone) functions of the TTV3620 are shown in Figure 26, along with the corresponding sequences of button presses.

Figure 26

Thomson-CSF TTV3620 Functions

Function	Key Presses	
1. Stop ("freeze")	STOP	
2. Play at programmed speed	>	
3. Play in reverse at programmed speed	<	
4. Scan forward	3	
5. Scan reverse	1	
6. Step forward	6	
7. Step reverse	4	
8. Set program speed 30 fps = $0 < n < 7$ = 1/128th normal*	9	n
9. Set program speed to twice normal (60 fps)	2	
10. Frame display on	5	1
11. Frame display off	5	0
12. Audio channel 1 on	8	1
13. Audio channel 2 on	8	2
14. Audio off	8	0

*Speed in fps = $\dfrac{30}{2^n}$

7.

Developing Computer-Controlled, Interactive Videodiscs

At first glance, it may not be apparent why placing the videodisc under the control of an external computer is a good idea. There has not been much of a rush to computerize *existing* media systems, such as film projectors, or tape recorders, so why should the videodisc be different? The principal reason for computer control is to enable the media device to be used as a component of a larger media system. There have been a number of special-purpose projectors and tape recorders that were designed to provide computer-control capabilities, but they have remained highly specialized machines, because the media formats were not themselves designed for computer access, and the mechanisms for reproduction were essentially mechanical. So the cost of retrofitting computer control added three to five times the cost of a simple player. From its inception, the optical videodisc has been designed with computer control as a desired mode of operation. Each frame is digitally numbered, and the control of the playback mechanism is accomplished by a series of electronic servomechanisms. Adding external control is merely a matter of inserting a few electronic impulses into an already existing electronic circuit.

Looking at the question from another angle, we see that the videodisc has a lot more capacity and flexibility than any previous media device. If there were a slide projector that could hold 54,000 slides, it would require computer control too! A third reason for computer control is that videodisc players are capable of operating so rapidly that a human can have a hard time keeping up with them, especially if they are performing a complex sequence of slow-motion and step-motion functions.

The two industrial players, the DiscoVision PR7820, and the Thomson-CSF TTV3620, can do essentially the same things under computer control—with two important exceptions: The TTV3620 can access 100,000 frames without turning the disc over; it just looks through the disc, by shifting focus to the other disc surface. On the PR7820, the disc must be unloaded, stopped, turned over, and reloaded (brought back up to speed and positioned under the laser beam) to get to the second set of 50,000 frames.

The second exception is the type of "conversation" that the machines have with their host computers; the TTV3620 uses a standard IEEE 488 interface protocol that allows the computer to interrogate the player to find out what it thinks it is doing, and where (what frame number) it thinks it is. In contrast, the PR7820 thinks of the computer as just another remote-control unit, a keyboard that gives it commands, but never "listens" to what is going on inside the player. So computers can tell the PR7820 what to do, but they cannot get the player to tell them whether or not it has done it yet.

Unlike the PR7820, the Thomson TTV3620 changes character when it is driven externally. The "mild-mannered home entertainment player" will now accept frame numbers and search them out, define up to 168 "chapters" by storing a sequence of frame numbers that mark chapter beginnings, tell the computer (when it asks) what frame it is at, and show what its status is (cassette in position, player loaded, searching, etc.). All of this is in addition to the commands available from the keyboard, except for the "scan-forward"

and "scan-reverse" commands. The TTV3620 can communicate a bit faster than the PR7820; it can operate at 30
characters per second, while 13 characters per second is tops
for the DVA unit. This higher speed, plus the ability to store
chapter boundaries, compensates for the lack of "stand-
alone" program storage capabilities. Notice that the
TTV3620 does not have an "auto-stop" command; with a
two-way interface, the computer can find out what frame the
player has reached, and issue a "stop" command when the
player has played as far as it is going to go. There are
advantages to both methods; with "auto-stop" on the
PR7820, you know the precise frame that the player will
freeze at every time. But your computer will have to do some
calculating to estimate *when* the player has stopped, because
the player won't tell it. With the Thomson two-way interface,
the computer does not have to calculate, it just asks. Of
course, when the desired frame comes along, it has to be
ready with the "stop" command. If it is a bit late, there is
likely to be some overshoot.

Computers and videodiscs can interact in another way:
their video output signals can be combined on a single CRT
screen by synchronizing the two signals and mixing them. It
takes a bit of additional circuitry, but with combined output,
the computer can "point" to portions of the videodisc image,
or add text or subtitles to it. This combined output
technique can overcome some of the problems of frequent
changes in the content (changes in rate structures, dates,
dollar amounts); the general, invariant material is put on the
videodisc, and the specific variable information is programmed into the computer and added to the display.

With the availability of these industrial videodisc players,
we have the opportunity to develop a new type of interactive
instructional delivery system. Now that the videodisc and
microcomputer are available, the production procedures,
including the authoring of good interactive courseware,

become more urgent. The problem is no longer one of media hardware availability. These two new technologies (videodisc and microcomputer) have essentially solved the hardware problem. As these technologies gain wider use and acceptance, low-cost, individualized instruction will become more economically feasible than ever before. The main problem that now faces us is authoring good, high-quality, interactive courseware that really *works*. The authoring of such courseware requires special techniques, and they are still in the developmental stages. As we indicated in 1976 (Schneider, 1976):

> The major feasibility questions do not revolve around the videodisc technology, but around a still-infant instructional technology. To be really cost-effective, videodiscs must be stamped in reasonable numbers; and, therefore, a reasonable number of schools and students must agree to use them. This acceptance will not occur unless the material stamped on the disc really works, and works well. And, it is not likely to work well unless it was developed and tested by people who had a pretty good idea of how to do the job right the first time. Unfortunately, instructional developers of such caliber are very few in number. Most CAI courses have been developed as if they were to be given as class lectures, and as a result, they have not turned out to be much of a cognitive improvement over the class lectures that they were designed to replace.

Several universities and industrial corporations have begun to develop interactive courseware for videodiscs (Merrill and Bennion, 1979). Initially, to gain experience, several groups have produced videodiscs using a variety of existing film or videotape footage just for the purpose of learning the best procedures for videodisc mastering. Every organization that has had a videodisc pressed has learned something about specific problems and procedures. In this chapter, we hope to summarize the proper procedures for producing pre-mastering media for videodisc, and some of the attendant problems that have been encountered by various videodisc research groups.

The development of interactive videodiscs is accomplished in five phases. The first phase is *authoring*: the product of this phase is a script. The second phase is *production*: the product of this phase is an edited film or videotape pre-master. The third phase is the *videodisc mastering and replication*: the product of this phase is the completed videodisc. The fourth phase is *programming the computer*: the product of this phase is a set of floppy discs to be used in actual operation of the videodisc/microcomputer delivery system.

The last phase is the *marketing and distribution* of the finished product: the product of this phase is a return on the capital expended during the first four phases. Without this phase, it becomes more difficult to repeat the entire process.

Authoring

Authoring procedures for *linear* videodiscs will not be discussed in this book, because linear videodiscs are designed and scripted in essentially the same way that instructional films or videotapes have been designed and scripted for many years. However, even the mode of displaying linear motion material using videodisc offers the student new opportunities over traditional motion media. Merely having local control over motion (i.e., allowing the student to stop, slow down, or repeat short portions of the videodisc) has demonstrated the ability to "rejuvenate" existing training films when they are transferred to videodisc. In the case of programs that use slow-motion or repetition techniques extensively, the footage can be shortened and the same techniques can be implemented by programming the player.

With a videodisc, the individual student does not remain a passive observer, just a part of a group sitting in a darkened room, listening to a noisy projector. The experience of trying to take notes or to write down questions under such circumstances is hopelessly frustrating. With his or her own videodisc, the student can employ a set of learning strategies not possible with film or videotape, even when the program material is in a linear sequence. Similarly, an instructor can use the freeze-frame mode to stop the motion and answer questions, repeat a sequence, or skip over parts that are non-essential or irrelevant—controls that were never available in traditional film or tape media—even though the videodisc was designed to be used in a linear fashion.

The author of interactive videodisc courseware must understand the capabilities and limitations of the various videodisc/microcomputer systems. For example, courseware for the Magnavox 8000 consumer model can be interactive within certain limits by using two types of codes that this player can read from the disc: the chapter-stop and the auto-stop codes. First, the videodisc can be organized into chapters. During the mastering process, a special code can be placed in a band of 400 frames at the beginning of each chapter. When using the "SEARCH" mode in either the forward or reverse direction, the videodisc player will stop automatically on the first of these 400 frames to be encountered by the laser beam. The Pioneer VP-1000 will search for chapter codes the same way it searches for frames. Up to 85 chapter codes can be accommodated on each side of a videodisc.

Second, the videodisc can be encoded with any number of auto-stop codes that will automatically change the player from any of the motion modes to the freeze-frame mode whenever a coded frame is encountered. However, because the first 10,000 Magnavox 8000 players were not equipped with electronics to read the stop codes (or because the disc may be used on other models), it is necessary to place a two- to three-second "STOP MOTION" label in the frames just preceding the auto-stop code. After the student observes the "STOP MOTION" label, he or she must quickly touch the stop key. The player can then be stepped ahead manually to the frame designed for the auto-stop code (a menu, question, text, etc.). Students using players equipped with the auto-stop circuitry could ignore the "STOP MOTION" label.

The truly new and obviously desirable feature of the industrial/educational videodisc players is their ability to be driven by a microcomputer. Several brands of microcomputers have been successfully interfaced to both the PR7820 and TTV3620 players, and several institutions are currently developing interactive videodiscs to demonstrate this new capability (Merrill and Bennion, 1979). Under computer control, the industrial/educational videodisc player can search out any frame within a few seconds, play forward or reverse in any of the several motion modes, pause on any frame for a specified time interval, branch to any other location, change audio tracks, and perform any sequence for a specified number of times. Computer-generated text and graphics characters can either be superimposed on the television screen or placed on a separate computer display. The latter allows text or graphics to be viewed simultaneously with the scene on the television.

Several combinations of videodisc/microcomputer hardware and software configurations are possible, as we have illustrated in the preceding chapters. *First*, a remote-control unit can be used to manually load program steps into the internal memory in the PR7820 player using the "PRO-GRAM" key. *Second*, the PR7820 player can also receive a program from a computer floppy disc or cassette. After the program is loaded by the computer into the videodisc player's memory, the computer can be disconnected and the operator can run the program using only the remote controller. *Third*, if a digital program exists on the videodisc, then the program can be inserted into the PR7820 player's memory directly without using a computer. The player can then be operated by the use of the remote controller. These last two combinations eliminate the manual inputting task that is very tedious and error-prone. *Fourth*, with a computer properly interfaced to either the PR7820 or the Thomson-CSF TTV3620 videodisc player, programs running in the external computer can select motion sequences or still frames from the videodisc and at the same time present text or graphics either on the computer terminal or on the TV monitor. *Fifth*, these same programs could be stored on the videodisc during the mastering process and then unloaded from the videodisc into the *external* computer's memory. This would save the cost of separate digital program storage (no cassette or floppy disc is needed to store the external computer's program), but is offset by the restriction of not being able to change the program after the videodisc has been mastered.

The last two configurations allow the full computer memory and branching logic to be harnessed to the visual storage available on the videodisc, thus making a very flexible and powerful interactive delivery system. An unlimited variety of programs can be supported, as long as the computer storage capacity and the basic resolution constraints of the 525-line television display are observed.

Beyond understanding the fundamental capabilities and limitations that have been discussed above, the author of interactive videodisc courseware must make basic strategy decisions concerning the locus of control. Typically, computer-assisted instruction (CAI) has utilized two basic types of control: *system control* and *learner control*. Both types of control can be implemented on the videodisc/microcomputer delivery system. Under a *system control* approach, the courseware is designed to move the student through the course content in a predetermined sequence, or as determined by system algorithms for selection of frames. The system decides what to show the student next based on the student's past performance. (However, pacing is usually under student control.) Under a *learner control* approach, the courseware is designed to provide orienting information, options for presentation modes, options for difficulty level, options for sequence, and options for study strategies. Courseware can be designed to provide learner control if that is desired; or, portions of the courseware can be designed to provide system control. The videodisc can accommodate either strategy or a mixture of the two.

There are also design decisions that will determine the aesthetic appeal and the motivational impact of the finished product. It is unfortunate, but many instructional designers have been so conditioned by the poor-quality sound and the half-focused visuals found in run-of-the-mill tape-slide shows that they continue working to the quality levels of the old medium after they have switched to videodisc. Veterans from programmed instruction and computer-assisted instruction have a similar problem; they are so used to presenting content without sound, color, or motion (and sometimes without lower-case letters!) that they have to rediscover the appeal and the subtlety of expression that video and sound can provide. And, the difference is a large one; it is the difference between sending someone a telegram, and talking with him or her face to face. It makes possible the insertion of incidental humorous touches without being heavy-handed and without making the program any longer. It makes it possible to engage the student by making him or her a part of a "real-world" experience. As we try to exploit these differences, we find ourselves drawn toward student-controlled dynamic simulations, fantasy games, and synthetic instructors reminiscent of "HAL," the spaceship computer in the movie "2001." We believe that instructional programs that require immediate responses in an interactive learning environment provide challenge, involvement, and excitement not attainable in typical group instruction.

Authoring Forms and Procedures

This section describes some forms and procedures for

scripting interactive videodisc courseware. These procedures spring from the necessity to specify (1) motion sequences, (2) still frames, and (3) the manner of interaction or branching that are to be implemented on the videodisc/ microcomputer delivery system. Three forms that have been used individually for scripting films, CAI frames, and computer programs, respectively, can be combined for the purpose of scripting interactive videodisc courseware. These forms are called "storyboard," "grid frames," and "branching networks or flowcharts," respectively.

The *storyboard* form consists of two parts. A box on the left side is used to sketch rough line drawings or descriptions of a motion sequence. On the right side, the text of the audio message and/or a description of background sounds is written. Other instructions to the photographer or the director can be placed in the unused space. For convenience in binding, several storyboard forms can be combined on a single sheet of paper as illustrated in Figure 27. Notes for transition from a motion sequence to a series of still frames can be included in the left boxes.

The *grid frames* are used for message layout of still frames that are to appear either on the computer display or on the TV screen. The usual capacity of computer displays is 80 x 24 characters, but it is advisable to use only a third of the capacity. For television, a maximum of about 35 characters per line should not be exceeded, due to poor TV resolution. The grid frames can be easily constructed on graph paper by placing a border around an area of 30 to 35 squares horizontally by 12 to 15 squares vertically (see Figure 28). The author then uses the enclosed area to design the still-frame message by placing characters in adjacent squares. This format forces the author to restrict the number of characters so that each character will be large enough for good resolution on the TV screen. Still frames should not look like pages of text. They should be similar to good

Figure 27

Storyboard Form

STORYBOARD   FILE _____
                                                  PAGE ___ OF __

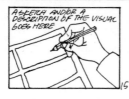

A SKETCH AND/OR A DESCRIPTION OF THE VISUAL GOES HERE

THE AUDIO MESSAGE IS WRITTEN VERBATIM IN THIS SPACE. IT CAN BE NEATLY HANDWRITTEN OR TYPED. IT MUST BE COMPLETE INCLUDING SUCH INDICATIONS FOR VOCALIZATION AS PAUSES (PAUSE) OR EXCLAMATIONS (EXCITEDLY), ETC. (YAWN).

| 1 |

15

THIS LINE SEPARATES THE AUDIO FROM INSTRUCTIONS TO THE PRODUCTION TEAM WHICH

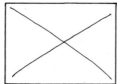

MAY EXTEND INTO THE NEXT BOX IF NEEDED. | X |
WHEN THIS HAPPENS THE BOX TO THE LEFT SHOULD BE MARKED WITH A LARGE X AS SHOWN
                    ALSO PUT AN X HERE
ALTERNATELY, IF MORE THAN ONE VISUAL BOX IS NEEDED THEN THE AUDIO MESSAGE BOX SHOULD BE LEFT BLANK.

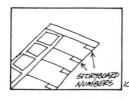

STORYBOARD NUMBERS

A SERIAL NUMBER FOR EACH STORYBOARD SEQUENCE SHOULD BE ENTERED IN THE UPPER RIGHT CORNER OF THE AUDIO MESSAGE BOX

| 2 |

10

    PUT THE STORY BOARD NUMBER HERE
PUT AN ESTIMATE OF TIME (IN SECONDS) THAT EACH MOTION SEQUENCE SHOULD OCCUPY ON THE VIDEO-DISC

STOP MOTION
_____
Still Frames 2
3, 4, 5, 6

INSERT THE STILL FRAME NUMBER IN THE VISUAL BOX PRECEDED BY A "STOP MOTION" LABEL WHEN AUTHORING FOR THE CONSUMER MODEL ONLY. REMEMBER THAT THE STILL FRAMES SHOULD BE NUMBERED CONSECUTIVELY WITHIN SEGMENTS

| 3 |
| S2-6 |

ENTER THE STILL FRAME NUMBER BELOW THE STORY BOARD NUMBER AS SHOWN HERE ———

Figure 28

Grid Frames

Frame No. *31* Code *Q3*

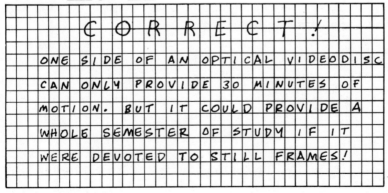

```
QUESTION: (MARK WRONG STATEMENT)
ONE SIDE OF A VIDEODISC:
1. CAN STORE 54000 STILL FRAMES.
               /O
2. CONTAINS 10   PITS OR MORE.
3. CAN BE USED FOR A MIRROR.
4. CAN PROVIDE 2 HOURS OF MOTION.
```

Frame No. *32* Code *FB4*

```
        C O R R E C T !
ONE SIDE OF AN OPTICAL VIDEODISC
CAN ONLY PROVIDE 30 MINUTES OF
MOTION. BUT IT COULD PROVIDE A
WHOLE SEMESTER OF STUDY IF IT
WERE DEVOTED TO STILL FRAMES!
```

overhead transparencies with lots of space between the lines. Space on the computer display does not cost anything. Only the characters "cost," by using space in memory.

Branching networks or flowcharts are used to describe the branching options allowed in an interactive videodisc program. A compact numbering scheme is needed to label where the still frames are to be inserted on the storyboard and to develop these branching networks or flowcharts. Any alphanumeric system that is internally consistent can be used. A sample of some of the symbols that could be used in scripting follows:

Scripting Symbol	Interpretation
SB14	Storyboard Sequence #14
SM	Stop Motion Message
Q5	Question #5
R5	Response #5
FB4	Feedback #4
UM2	Unit Map #2
LM3	Lesson Map #3
MU1	Menu for Unit 1
ML2	Menu for Lesson 2

The author should develop a complete list of symbols and use them consistently throughout the script. An example of how these symbols can also be used to develop branching networks is illustrated in Figure 29. Branching networks provide a "road map" of all of the lesson components, showing their relationship to each other. They are also needed during the programming phase to communicate the author's courseware design to the programmer.

The script for an interactive videodisc is merely an ordered collection of the three forms discussed above: storyboards, grid frames, and branching networks. For most educational materials, these three forms will be adequate to describe the content and the presentation strategy to be implemented on an interactive videodisc/microcomputer delivery system.

Another type of scripting form has been developed that

Figure 29

Branching Networks

a. Motion Sequences with Multiple Choice Questions:

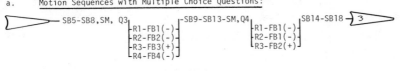

b. Unit Menu leading to Lesson Menus:

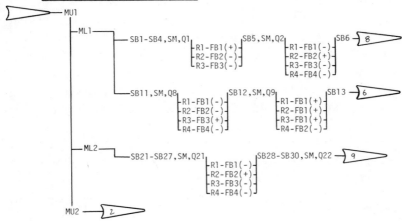

c. Motion Sequence Ending in a Series of Questions:

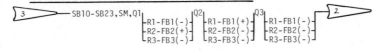

combines the features of all three of these forms (see Figure 30). This form may be more useful for discs where motion sequences are short and where many opportunities for branching are required. This form has four main parts, used to describe motion, audio, still frame, and branching addresses. Three other parts on the form are used to assign a serial number to the form, record a short title, and record the previous form in the script that led to this form. These scripting forms allow the author to try out the branching logic by "playing computer" and thus permit colleagues to visualize the program as a student would see it before the program is produced.

A fully developed script is a valuable interim product that can be reviewed, analyzed, and evaluated by academic departments, funding agencies, and potential publishers. The script can be developed at low cost by content specialists working individually or as part of an instructional development team. Developing a script is a valuable experience that helps the author finalize all instructional sequences, question frames, and branching logic ready for production without having any programming experience. It also allows the instructional development team to visualize the production and programming tasks required to transfer the script into the final product; an exciting, interactive, instructional videodisc.

Production

Since videodiscs are mastered from videotape, one would suppose that videotape would be the best medium for production of motion sequences. This is not always true, as we shall see when we examine one small aspect of the actual television (videotape) process. A video camera scans each image twice, producing two fields that are combined to form one frame. The first field is separated in time by 1/60 of a second from the next field. Consequently, when dynamic

Figure 30

Scripting Cards

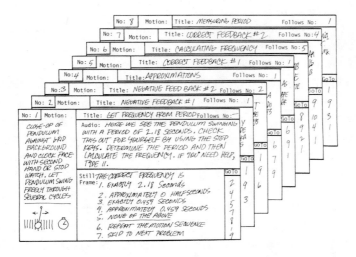

motion (a golf swing, for example) is being videotaped, the position of moving objects (the golf club and the golfer's arms) is displaced slightly from field one to field two. Under normal television viewing conditions, this displacement is never observed because the persistence of the eye integrates and smooths over such motion. However, when these fields are transferred to videodisc, and the freeze-frame mode is used, then the images on each of the two fields are seen over and over again, and the displacement between the positions of the images appears as a rapidly oscillating image (the golf club might wave back and forth rapidly). Imagine the effect of such flickering on a class of juvenile athletes if a videodisc designed to display tumbling techniques were produced using videotape. As the instructor tries to display the proper technique for cartwheels, the legs of the upturned model flicker whenever a freeze frame is used. The moral to this story is: Whenever a videodisc is designed to contain dynamic motion and is to be used in the freeze-frame mode, always use *film* for the original production medium. When film frames are transferred to videotape, two identical video fields are generated from each film frame, and when these two fields are shown together as a freeze frame, the image will not flicker. Alternatively, a rotating-shutter video camera can be used, but finding this type of equipment is difficult.

The post-production process for producing a pre-master tape or film for interactive videodiscs presents some unique problems to producers and directors who have been producing linear film or videotape. In principle, the sequences on an interactive videodisc can be arranged in any order, because the computer can rearrange the order for actual presentation. Gone is the need for fades, transitions, and other scene-bridging production techniques. In fact, some videodisc producers recommend throwing in everything that may ever have any possible use. Hundreds of still frames can be added in random order, and the computer programmer can "straighten it all out later." However, we feel that careful design and planning of the order of sequences on the disc will make the programmer's task easier, and improve the performance of the finished product by minimizing search times.

Preparing the audio tracks is very simple with a videotape master, because the video formats make provision for two audio tracks. What you put on those tracks is what you will hear on your disc. The audio quality is excellent in terms of both frequency response and low background noise, so listen carefully to your master tape; connect the audio channels to a good sound system and check the levels, the frequency equalization, the noise level, and the channel balance (if you are recording stereophonically). Remember that the videodisc players do not have volume controls, so the levels cannot be "tweaked up" later.

If you are mastering from film with a single optical or magnetic soundtrack, that will work nicely, but if you want two sound channels, they will have to be recorded on 35mm magnetically-coated film (also known as "full-coat"). DVA prefers a three-track format, but they can cope with other configurations.

If your disc is going to load the player's memory when it is played, the program to be loaded must be written beforehand, and should be checked very carefully by manually loading the program and trying it out with an existing disc. If your program will be searching for one unique frame, your starting frame must be clearly marked, and your frame numbering must be "right on." Sometimes, if the disc is not completely full, you can buy some "insurance" by putting on three to five copies of every still frame.

Videodisc Mastering and Replication

Before you prepared your master, you had already contacted the people who were going to make your discs, told them what format you were going to use, how long the program was supposed to run, and when you would be ready to roll. Programming procedures and forms should have been mentioned, if that was being contemplated. Now, months later, you are ready to have your show transferred to disc. In the case of a programmed disc, the manufacturer will encode your program on the master tape. It will go right up front, on the second audio track. Then your master will be transferred to 2" helical videotape. The frame numbers will be generated at the same time, and encoded into the first part of each frame. Chapter numbers and stop codes also go in, if you specify where you want them. The completed 2" tape is checked and re-checked, and then sent to the transfer room for mastering. The rest of the process is described in Chapter 5. If you are making a programmed disc, you can ask for a check disc, to verify the synchronization of program code and frame numbers. Naturally, these little extras for the programmed discs add up: DVA charges an extra ten percent for mastering, and an extra 20 percent for the discs themselves. If your disc has a long program of multiple program dumps, the prices will be increased again. Program or no program, DVA wants a minimum order of 50 replicated discs per master. This is quite reasonable for any kind of production run, but some of us researchers are going to be buying a lot of $10 Frisbees.

At this writing (mid-1980), it takes about 45 working days for mastering and replication. As more videodisc plants are built, that time will probably shrink 30 percent to 50 percent.

Programming the Computer

Programming the videodisc can occur at three levels: (1) using only the PR7820 remote controller, (2) using an external computer to load program steps into the PR7820 videodisc memory, and (3) using an external computer to control the videodisc in an interactive mode. The first two levels have been discussed previously. A manual has been prepared that describes the procedures involved in programming the PR7820 videodisc player using the remote controller (Morehead and Schneider, 1980).

The second level of programming allows the same type of programs that are loaded manually to be loaded automatically by a computer. The advantage is that the manual inputting task, which is slow and error-prone, is eliminated. For example, we have developed one program of about 700 steps that can be loaded without errors into the videodisc player memory in about 80 seconds using the computer. Manual inputting of this program requires at least 30 minutes and usually contains several errors that take additional time to find and to correct.

The third level of programming makes use of the interactive capabilities of the computer. In order for this level of programming to be possible, there are several subroutines that must be developed. For example, the transfer of commands (search, stop, play, etc.—there are 34) must meet the needs of both the author/programmer *and* the hardware. These commands are first entered as three-letter mnemonic commands (SRC = Search, STP = Stop, PLA = Play, etc.) so that they are more easily remembered by the programmer. However, the videodisc will only accept a string of numbers representing the eight-bit numbers that drive the videodisc. Hence, a subroutine to transform input commands to output numbers is needed. Many other subroutines are needed and must be developed to facilitate the programming task. These subroutines form building blocks for the full-scale program. A partial list of subroutines that we have developed thus far is presented in Table 8.

With these and other subroutines, the computer can provide the following types of displays and interactions: (1) input commands to the videodisc microprocessor, (2) put up text or graphics on a separate CRT or on the television terminal, (3) receive responses through the keyboard or other devices, such as touch panels, joysticks, etc., and process these responses, and (4) control other peripheral devices, such as an auxiliary audiocassette player/recorder, a printer, or a speech synthesizer. With these tools, the programmer can assemble a plethora of presentation and interactive strategies.

It is important that the computer programs be kept in an erasable form (floppy disc) during program development and early stages of evaluation. After the program has been perfected and tried out extensively, it can be transferred to a second pre-master tape and coded on a second-generation videodisc for wide-scale distribution. We recommend that a second-generation videodisc be considered only after considerable experience has been gained with each videodisc program.

Marketing and Distribution

The marketing and distribution of interactive videodiscs

Table 8

Subroutines

---

1. *Videodisc transfer*
   a. Timing loop
   b. Command recognition
   c. Mnemonic to output bit transfer

2. *Audiocassette driver*
   a. Reset counter and memory to zero
   b. Load counter
   c. Read counter
   d. Load status
   e. Interrogate status

3. *Menu display*
   a. Unpacking (short, long, overlap) synchronized with file building program
   b. Print
   c. Execution

4. *Student Response*
   a. "Continue" option
   b. Previous scene option   These routines
   c. Spanish and English option   also use the above
   d. End program option   in some fashion.
   e. Question branching
       i reprint the question
       ii retrieve answer from disc
       iii print answer
   f. Reprint instructions

---

has been a possibility for less than a year. Marketing opportunities are increasing as more videodisc players are sold. For many years, these markets will be tied to major companies, universities, or other large organizations, including the military services, who may purchase large numbers of videodisc players and computers that are capable of using interactive videodiscs. We expect that each organization that uses this new method of instruction will at first either rely on its own video or film production facilities or establish close ties to other highly qualified studios to get videodiscs produced. Assistance from videodisc manufacturers, through their client support centers, will be given for educational videodisc program development. In June, 1980, MCA, North American Philips (parent of Magnavox), and U.S. Pioneer Electronics announced the formation of a partnership called Optical Programming Associates (OPA) to help software producers create videodiscs. OPA wishes to assist in the creation of videodiscs designed for education and training that will show off the optical videodisc system's special features, such as frame access, motion control, and two-channel sound.

If OPA is able to sell a large number of a few educational videodiscs, they may be able to provide a "pipeline" for marketing additional interactive videodiscs.

We expect that many organizations may join together to form consortia to sell interactive videodiscs to each other. Some organizational structures already exist within certain professional societies that have been distributing media to their members in other formats. The legal and medical professions, for example, are highly organized in this manner and will undoubtedly provide interactive videodiscs to members when both the economic and educational advantages of this new technology have been clearly demonstrated.

Educational institutions are generally slow to accept innovations in instructional processes, and interactive videodiscs will probably be marketed to these institutions as if they were textbooks. For example, McGraw-Hill, a large textbook supplier, has already funded a pilot videodisc for biology.

Who will market videodiscs for education and training? Professional societies? Textbook publishers? Television producers? We do not know the answer, but we suspect that the most successful group will be the one who can reach the broadest market and take full advantage of the lower costs that high-volume videodisc replication can offer.

8.

Future Trends

As a commercial product, videodiscs are in their infancy. In fact, some of the players have yet to emerge from the "delivery room." The most crucial improvements will be in the area of replicating discs. By the beginning of 1981, we expect to see three firms offering transfer and replication services. The largest will continue to be DiscoVision Associates (DVA). This firm is currently building several new plants to greatly increase production capacity. At the same time, improvements are being made in the replication process so that fewer discs will be rejected because of molding defects. Other refinements in the mastering process will make the production of extended play discs (60 minutes of video per side) more common.

The other major area of improvement will be in the videodisc players. The large and relatively costly helium-neon gas laser will be replaced by a solid-state laser. This light source is so small that it can be integrated into the assembly that holds the objective lens. This refinement ought to reduce player cost by $100 to $200, and provide some improvement in access time, better resistance to variations in temperature, and an even more rugged and durable optical assembly.

The players will also improve in their ability to communicate with external computers. Already, the Thomson-CSF player has an interface that is directly compatible with virtually all of the eight-bit microcomputer systems. Tomorrow's interfaces will be much faster at transferring data and will allow data transfers to the on-board memory (direct memory access). Internally, improvements in the search algorithms that are used by the on-board microprocessor for locating specific frames will result in faster and more reliable access times.

Philips has already announced a new type of videodisc player. It is a digital videodisc system that allows purchasers to record their own data discs. The digital discs will hold approximately ten gigabits (10×10^9) and will resemble an "air sandwich": a layer of plastic, a metalized layer, an air space, a metalized layer, and a second layer of clear plastic. The air layer will provide a "miniature cleanroom" so that the optically critical surface, the metalized layer, will be free of contamination. As the digital information is being burned into the metal surface, a second (much less powerful) laser beam reads the information back, and compares it with the information being written. If there are any discrepancies, the track can be "scratched out" by writing a special code in front of the data block, and then the data are written again on a new track. The developers see this disc as being used as a massive "scratch pad" memory. Information will be written on it and then accessed for read-out as needed. When the disc becomes full, the tracks which still contain needed data can be transferred to a new disc, and the scratch memory process resumes on the new disc. Because of the different construction, digital discs will not be capable of replication. So this system will be for local storage, rather than widespread communication. Not to be outdone, RCA Advanced Technology Laboratories are developing a one-hundred disc data "jukebox," using optical videodisc technology.

Although no marketing announcements have yet been made, MCA and IBM have been working on a high-resolution document storage and retrieval system that will rival today's best microfilm systems. With this system, each frame is stored as a concentric circle on the disc, instead of being one revolution of the continuous helix. Once the user locates the desired frame, the optical head will continue to track that frame without requiring a reset pulse at each revolution. The result should be a simpler, more reliable player that is easier to align.

Videodiscs have some especially attractive properties for very long-term storage of information. Georges Broussaud of Thomson-CSF speaks of the micropits on the videodisc as "micro-hieroglyphics." The microglyphs represent a physical deformation of a material surface, just as the ancient Egyptian and Assyrian scribes marked clay tablets. As a result, they will last much, much longer than ink on paper or a silver halide chemical complex. Brossard has estimated that if the metal stamper from which the plastic videodisc is made were stored in an inert atmosphere (e.g., krypton gas), the limiting physical factor would be the rate at which metallic ions would diffuse from the surface of the stamper into the inert gas. The diffusion of the informational layer would take approximately 50 thousand years, according to his calculations.

In Japan, Hitachi, Ltd. has been working on a holographic videodisc. The disc contains a string of one-millimeter-square holograms. Each hologram is actually three separate images, one each for brightness, color, and sound. A 12-inch disc would rotate at six rpm and store a half-hour program.

A newly-formed subsidiary of Atlantic Richfield called ARDEV is developing an optical videodisc that is made from photographic film. The principal advantage of their system is the ease of disc replication; any of their discs can be used as a photographic negative to contact-print a copy. The film stock is much more expensive than molded plastic discs, but for small runs, it is more economical than electroplating metal stampers.

There are a large number of alternative systems that are under intense development. In view of this, we should look at today's videodisc systems as just instances of a large class of extremely high-density information storage and retrieval systems that will be available in the future. With the exception of the imaginative work being done by a few research groups, the educational applications of this technology lag far behind the technological capabilities.

The trend that *we* will be watching most closely is the response of our fellow educators to these new capabilities. Will they develop their own production and distribution networks through professional societies, etc., or, will they wait for publishers' representatives to sell them discs at retail? Will educators spend enough time with the new equipment to learn how to use the programming and motion-control features? Or, will they be satisfied with linear programs that cost less per copy and last longer? Are educators willing to restructure their roles and their institutions to take maximum advantage of new technologies?

If educators do not rise to the challenge, will other enterprises, such as calculator and computer manufacturers, entertainment producers, or even cable-TV operators, step in and provide new educational alternatives? We may not be able to answer these questions for another ten or 20 years; but we are no longer willing to bet on "business as usual" as the most likely outcome.

References

Bennion, J.L., "Possible Applications of Optical Videodiscs to Individualized Instruction," *Technical Report No. 10*, Institute for Computer Uses in Education, Brigham Young University, February, 1974.

Bennion, J.L., and E.W. Schneider, "Interactive Videodisc Systems for Education," *Journal of the SMPTE*, 84(12), December, 1975, pp. 949-953.

Bolt, Richard A., *Spatial Data-Management System*, Massachusetts Institute of Technology, 1979, 60 pp.

Bounhius, G., and P. Burgstede, "The Optical Scanning System of the Philips VLP Record Player," *Philips Technical Review*, 33(7), 1973, pp. 186-189.

Broadbent, K.D., "Review of the MCA DiscoVision System," *Journal of the SMPTE*, 83, July, 1974, pp. 554-559.

Carter, Clyde N., and Maurice J. Walker, "Costs of Instructional TV and Computer-Assisted Instruction in Public Schools," *The Schools and the Challenge of Innovation*, McGraw-Hill Book Company, New York, 1969, pp. 320-341.

Chapman, D. *Design for ETV: Planning for Schools in Television*, Educational Facilities Laboratories, New York, 1960.

Compaan, K., and P. Kramer, "The Philips VLP System," *Philips Technical Review*, 33(7), 1973, pp. 178-180.

Dickopp, Gerhard, and Horst Redlich, "Design Simplicity Cuts Costs for German Color-Video Disk System," *Electronics*, September, 1973, pp. 93-99.

Hrbek, G.W., "An Experimental Optical Videodisc Playback System," *Journal of the SMPTE*, 83, July, 1974, pp. 580-582.

Janssen, P.J.M., and P.E. Day, "Control Mechanisms in the Philips VLP Record Player," *Philips Technical Review*, 33(7), 1973, pp. 190-193.

Jerome, J.A., and E.M. Kaczorowshi, "Film-Based Videodisc System," *Journal of the SMPTE*, 83, July, 1974, pp. 560-563.

Leith, Emmett N., "White-Light Holograms," *Scientific American*, October, 1976, pp. 80-95.

Leveridge, Leo L., "The Potential of Interactive Optical Videodisc Systems for Continuing Education, *Educational and Industrial Television*," 11(4), April, 1979, pp. 35-38.

Lewis, Philip. *Educational Television Guidebook*. McGraw-Hill, New York, 1961.

Merrill, Paul F., and Junius L. Bennion, "Videodisc Technology in Education: The Current Scene," *NSPI Journal*, November, 1979, pp. 18-26.

Monaco, James, *How to Read a Film*, Oxford University Press, New York, 1977, 502 pp.

Morehead, William H., and Edward W. Schneider, *Operating and Programming for the MCA DiscoVision Industrial Model Videodisc Players*, David O. McKay Institute of Education, Provo, 1980, 35 pp.

Pfannkuch, R., "Characteristics of the Videodisc Systems," *Journal of the SMPTE*, 83, July, 1974, pp. 580-586.

"The RCA 'SelectaVision' Videodisc System," *Information Display*, May, 1976, pp. 20-23.

Roberts, M., and Associates. *The Videocassette and CATV Newsletter*. April, 1979, pp. 1-2.

Schneider, E.W., "Videodiscs, or the Individualization of Instructional Television," *Educational Technology*, May, 1976, pp. 53-58. Reprinted in *Instructional Television: Status and Directions*, Educational Technology Publications, Englewood Cliffs, New Jersey, 1977, pp. 133-145.

Schneider, E.W., "Applications of Videodisc Technology to Individualized Instruction," *Computers and Communication,* Academic Press, New York, 1977, pp. 313-325.

Silberman, Charles E., *Crisis in the Classroom,* Random House, New York, 1970, 350 pp.

Snyder, Ross H., "Video Tape Recorder Uses Revolving Head," *Electronics,* 30(8), August, 1957, p. 138.

Van der Bussche, W. *et al.,* "Signal Processing in the Philips VLP System," *Philips Technical Review,* 33(7), 1973, pp. 181-185.

Videodisc Design/Production Group, University of Nebraska-Lincoln, 1(1), August, 1979.

"Videodisc Update: Instruction and Training," *The Videoplay Report,* C.S. Tepfer Publishing Co., Inc., 8(14), July 10, 1978, pp. 57-60.

Willis, Barry D., "Formats for the Videodisc—What Are the Options?," *Educational and Industrial Television,* May, 1979, pp. 36-38.

Winslow, K. "A Videodisc in Your Future," *Educational and Industrial TV,* May, 1977, pp. 21-22.

Zwaneveld, E., "An Audiovisual Producer/User's View of Videodisc Technology," *Journal of the SMPTE,* July, 1974, pp. 583-594.

Appendix A

Analysis of the Educational Potential
of the First DiscoVision Catalog

I. Instructional programs, by topic.

Art
Art Awareness Collection from the National Gallery
The Art Conservator
LeCorbusier

Cuisine
Julia Child (French)
    Boeuf Bourguignon
    The Omelette Show
    Quiche Lorraine & Co.
    To Roast a Chicken
Theonis Marks (Greek)
    Baklava/Orange Sweets
    Cheese Triangles/Egg Lemon Soup
    Moussaka/Baked Spaghetti
    Spinach Pie/Dolmathes
Franco and Margaret Romagnoli (Italian)
    Abruzzi Specialties
    From Florence with Love
    Made in Milan

Elementary Education
    Forgive & Forget/Thank You, Thank You
    Magic Moments
    Math That Counts
    Money in the Marketplace/Choosing What to Buy
    Silent Safari

Health & Fitness
  CPR & Choking: To Save a Life
  Nobody's Victim II
  Smoking: How to Stop
  Total Fitness in 30 Minutes a Week
  Venereal Disease: The Hidden Epidemic

Music
The Bolero by Ravel, with Zubin Mehta
Elton John at Edinburgh

Natural History
African Animals, with Jane Goodall
  The Baboons of Gourlie
  The Hyena Story
  Lions of Serengheti
  The Wild Dogs of Africa
Archaeological Dating/The Big Dig
Ecology (Barry Commoner)
Silent Safari (East African Game Reserves)
The Solar System/The Universe
The Undersea World of Jacques Cousteau
  The Coral Divers of Corsica
  Octopus-Octopus
  The Singing Whales
  The Sleeping Sharks of Yucatan
  The Smile of the Walrus
  A Sound of Dolphins
  The Tragedy of the Red Salmon
  The Unsinkable Sea Otter
What Makes It Rain?/Storms: The Restless Atmosphere

Needlecraft
Designing Needlepoint/Geometric Needlepoint
Satin Stitch/Chains

Religion and Moral Values
Forgive & Forget/Thank You, Thank You
The Guide
A Light Shines in the Darkness
The Making of a Torah/A Portrait of Jewish Marriage
Mission to Love: The Call of Confirmation
The Way Home
Who Is God? Where Is God?/God's World, Our World

Social Studies
The Amish
Women at Work

Sports Instruction
Basketball with Bill Foster & Gail Goodrich
Better Tennis in 30 Minutes
Champions Never Quit (with Bart Starr)
Gene Littler's Golf
If You Can Walk (Cross-Country Skiing)/Listen to the Mountains
Sentinel: The West Face
Skateboard Safety
Swimming: Breast Stroke & Butterfly
Swimming: Freestyle & Backstroke

II. Sports performances; not "how to" programs, but they offer learning by example.

Boxing
Ali vs. Folley/Ali vs. Williams
Louis vs. Conn I/Louis vs. Conn II
Marciano vs. Wolcott/Marciano vs. Moore
Robinson vs. Graziano/Robinson vs. LaMotta

Football (National Football League)
Catch It if You Can
Gamebreakers
The Runners
They Call It Pro Football
Trials and Triumphs
Young, Old, and Bold

Skiing
Mammoth Mountain
The Moebus Flip
Ski Racer
Winterwings

Tennis
In Pursuit of No. 6 (Jimmy Connors, Dick Stockton)
Killer Instinct (Brian Gottfried, Buillermo Vilas)

III. Film versions of theatrical productions; useful in English and drama classes at secondary and continuing education levels.

Animal Crackers
   musical play by George S. Kaufman *et al.*
Anne of the Thousand Days
   play by Maxwell Anderson
A Delicate Balance
   play by Edward Albee
Destry Rides Again
   Broadway musical
Jesus Christ Superstar
   rock opera, book by Tim Rice
Luther
   play by John Osborne
The Man in the Glass Booth
   play by Edward Anhalt
Sweet Charity
   Broadway musical, based on film *Nights of Cabiria*, by Federico Fellini
Three Sisters
   play by Anton Chekhov

IV. Dance; excellent examples for a modern dance class

Acrobats of God	Martha Graham Dance Co.
Cortege of Eagles	Martha Graham Dance Co.
Seraphic Dialog	Martha Graham Dance Co.

V. Orchestra; the "chemistry" between conductor and musicians
The Bolero by Ravel
   conducted by Zubin Mehta

VI. Historical vignettes; these films range from pure documentaries to pure historical fiction. In the latter case, only a few scenes may be appropriate to illustrate an historical epoch.

Film	*Epoch*
Anne of the Thousand Days	English History
Luther	Reformation
MacArthur	World War II
The Man in the Glass Booth	World War II
Midway	World War II
Shenandoah	Civil War
The World at War	
The Bomb	Hiroshima
Bonzai	Pearl Harbor
Genocide	Nazi concentration camps
Morning	D-Day

VII. Rewards for reading; these films are all based on published books. Some of the books are immortal classics, others are not. But all of them could be used to reward readers when they complete the book. Class discussion of a book may be much more lively if it starts off with comparisons of the film interpretation with the individual reader's impressions. An * marks books that are especially suitable for children.

* *Almost Angels,* story by R.A. Stemmle
   Andromeda Strain, novel by Michael Crichton
   Back Street, from a story by Fannie Huest
   The Bingo Long Traveling All-Stars & Motor Kings, novel by William Brasher
   The Birds, short story by Daphne DuMaurier
   Bullitt, from *Mute Witness,* novel by Robert L. Pike
   The Choirboys, novel by Joseph Wambaugh
* *Cyborg: The Six Million Dollar Man,* novel by Martin Caiden
   The Day of the Jackal, novel by Frederick Forsyth
   Deliverance, novel by James Dickey
   Destry Rides Again, novel by Max Brand
   Diary of a Mad Housewife, novel by Sue Kaufman
   Dracula, novel by Brian Stoker
   East of Eden, novel by John Steinbeck
   The Eiger Sanction, novel by Travanian
   Family Plot from the *Rainbird Pattern,* by Victor Canning
* *Francis, the Talking Mule,* novel by David Stern
   Frankenstein, novel by Mary Shelley
   Frenzy, from *Goodbye Piccadilly, Farewell Leicester Square,* by Arthur La Bern
   Gray Lady Down from *Event 1000,* by David Lavallee
* *Greyfriars Bobby,* story by Eleanor Atkinson
   The Incredible Shrinking Man, novel by Richard Matheson
   Jaws, novel by Peter Benchley
* *Kidnapped,* story by Robert Lewis Stevenson
   To Kill a Mockingbird, novel by Harper Lee
* *The Littlest Outlaw,* story by Larry Lansburgh
   Lonely Are the Brave, novel by Edward Abbey
   Looking for Mr. Goodbar, novel by Judith Rossner
   Love Story, novel by Erich Segal
* *Miracle of the White Stallions,* from the book *The Dancing White Horses of Vienna,* by Col. Alois Podhajsky
* *The Moon Spinners,* book by Mary Stewart
   The Other Side of the Mountain, from *A Long Way Up,* by E.G. Valen
* *Perri,* novel by Felix Satten

* *The Prince and the Pauper*, story by Mark Twain
  Psycho, novel by Robert Black
* *The Railway Children*, novel by E. Nesbit
  The Seven Per-Cent Solution, novel by Nicholas Meyer
  Slaughterhouse Five, novel by Kurt Vonnegut
* *The Slipper and the Rose*, musical version of *Cinderella*
* *Tom Sawyer*, story by Mark Twain

VIII. Film as an art form; these films can be used to illustrate discussions of directors, actors, styles, and techniques; with the stop-frame capabilities of the videodisc, animation and editing techniques can be viewed a frame at a time.

The Adventures of Chip 'n' Dale—Animation Techniques

Animal Crackers—Marx Brothers

At Home with Donald Duck—Animation Techniques

Back Street—Irene Dunne, Zasu Pitts

The Coyote's Lament—Animation Techniques

Double Indemnity—Billy Wilder, Dir.

Dracula—Bela Lugosi

East of Eden—Elia Kazan, Dir.; James Dean, Julie Harris, Raymond Massey

Fellini's Casanova—Federico Fellini, Dir.

Frankenstein—James Whale, Dir.; Boris Karloff

The Godfather—Francis Ford Coppola, Dir.; Marlon Brando, Al Pacino, James Caan

Going My Way—Bing Crosby, Barry Fitzgerald

If I Had a Million—W.C. Fields, Charlie Ruggles, Charles Laughton, Gary Cooper, Jack Oakie, Alison Skipworth, George Raft

The Incredible Shrinking Man—Special Effects

Kids Is Kids—Animation Techniques

Lonely Are the Brave—Kirk Douglas, Walter Matthau, George Kennedy, Carroll O'Connor

The Lost Weekend—Billy Wilder, Dir.; Ray Milland, Jane Wyman, Howard de Silva

On Vacation with Mickey Mouse and Friends—Animation Techniques

Psycho—Alfred Hitchcock, Dir.

Ruggles of Red Gap—Charles Laughton, Mary Boland, Charlie Ruggles, Zasu Pitts

The Ten Commandments—Cecil B. DeMille, Dir.; Charleton Heston, Yul Brynner, Anne Baxter, Edward G. Robinson, Yvonne DeCarlo *et al.*

Three Days of the Condor—Robert Redford, Faye Dunaway, Cliff Robertson, Max von Sydow

Three Sisters—Sir Lawrence Olivier, Dir.; Alan Bates, Sir Lawrence Olivier, Joan Plowright

What's Up, Doc?—Peter Bogdonovich, Dir.

The Wild Bunch—Sam Peckinpah, Dir.; William Holden, Ernest Borgnine, Robert Ryan

Appendix B

Commands for PR7820 Videodisc Player

The following commands, reprinted from Morehead and Schneider (1980), summarize the control capabilities provided by the industrial/educational model players. The abbreviations are the ones used by the McKay Institute Videodisc Project and have no "official" status. Having standard codes, though, greatly improves interpersonal communication. See pages 116 and 117.

Command	Abbr.	Function	Format	Example
AUDIO 1	AD1	Turns channel 1 sound on ("1") or off ("0").*	<"0" or "1"> AD1	0 AD1
AUDIO 2	AD2	Turns channel 2 sound on ("1") or off ("0").*	<"0" or "1"> AD2	1 AD2
AUTO STOP	ATP	Plays forward from current frame to the specified frame and stops.	<Frame number> ATP	2100 ATP
BRANCH	BRN	Allows a program to skip or repeat certain program steps.	<Pgm. step no.> BRN	0 BRN
DECREMENT REGISTER	DEC	Program repeats a given number of times.	<Register number> DEC	1 DEC [...BRN]
END	END	Takes player out of program mode.	END	END
FRAME DISPLAY	DIS	Turns frame display on ("1") or off ("0").*	<"0" or "1"> DIS	0 DIS
HALT	HLT	Stops the program.	HLT	HLT
INPUT	INP	Allows a choice.	< #of choices> INP	2 INP [...BRN] [...BRN]
PROGRAM	PGM	Puts videoplayer in program mode, starting at the specified step number.	<Pgm. step no.> PGM	0 PGM
RECALL	RCL	Recalls a given register.	<Register number> RCL	3 RCL
RUN	RUN	Used to run a program.	<Pgm. step no.> RUN	0 RUN
SEARCH	SRC	Locates a particular frame.	<Frame number> SRC	2100 SRC

*If the leading "0" or "1" is omitted, the function is "toggled," i.e., changes state.

Command	Abbr.	Function	Format	Example
SLOW MOTION, FWD	SLF	Plays forward in slow motion, starting at the current frame and stopping at the specified frame. The specified frame must be larger than the current frame.	\<Frame number\> SLF	2100 SLF
SLOW MOTION, REV	SLR	Plays in reverse in slow motion, starting at the current frame and stopping at the specified frame. The specified frame must be smaller than the current frame.	\<Frame number\> SLR	2100 SLR
STEP FORWARD	STF	Moves one frame forward.	STF	STF
STEP REVERSE	STR	Moves one frame backward.	STR	STR
STORE	STO	Stores a number in a previously-recalled register.	\<number\> STO	1 RCL 2100 STO
WAIT	WAT	Puts a pause in the program. (Use STOP key.)	\<#seconds x 10\> WAT	30 WAT
PLAY	PLA	Starts program running when using manual mode.	PLA	PLA
STOP	STP	Stops play in manual mode. Used for timed pause in program mode.	STP	STP
REJECT	REJ	Removes disc from play position and resets player's microprocessor.	REJ	REJ
CLEAR	CLR	Removes register display from screen. Aborts running program.	CLR	CLR

About the Authors

Edward W. Schneider is an Instructional Scientist on the staff of the David O. McKay Institute of Education and an Associate Professor of Instructional Science at Brigham Young University. While working on the development of the TICCIT computer-assisted instruction system, he became interested in the enhancements that videodisc technology could offer to computer-assisted instruction. He has made numerous presentations about educational applications of computers and video-discs to education at conferences sponsored by the National Science Foundation, the American Educational Research Association, the California Department of Education, and the U.S. Air Force.

Junius L. Bennion is also a staff member of the David O. McKay Institute of Education at Brigham Young University. As an Instructional Scientist, he is responsible for coordinating instructional improvements using new technology within the university. He became interested in videodisc technology as an improvement to computer-assisted instruction while working on the TICCIT project as a graduate student in instructional science. He has participated in several conferences to discuss and demonstrate interactive videodisc authoring procedures and products applied to education.